AF854866

INTERNATIONAL NARCOTICS CONTROL BOARD
ORGANE INTERNATIONAL DE CONTRÔLE DES STUPÉFIANTS
JUNTA INTERNACIONAL DE FISCALIZACIÓN DE ESTUPEFACIENTES

Psychotropic Substances
Substances psychotropes
Sustancias sicotrópicas

Statistics for 2023
Assessments of Annual
Medical and Scientific Requirements
for Substances in Schedules II, III and IV of the Convention
on Psychotropic Substances of 1971 for 2025

Statistiques pour 2023
Prévisions des besoins annuels
médicaux et scientifiques concernant
les substances des Tableaux II, III et IV de la Convention
sur les substances psychotropes de 1971 pour 2025

Estadísticas de 2023
Previsiones de las necesidades anuales
para fines médicos y científicos
de las sustancias de las Listas II, III y IV del Convenio
sobre Sustancias Sicotrópicas de 1971 para 2025

UNITED NATIONS
NATIONS UNIES
NACIONES UNIDAS
Vienna, 2025

E/INCB/2024/3

UNITED NATIONS PUBLICATION
Sales No.: T.25.XI.3
ISBN: 978-92-1-0034531
eISBN: 978-92-1-107123-8
ISSN 0253-9403
eISSN 2412-4656

CONTENTS

*The annexes are not included in the printed and electronic versions of the present publication, but are available on the website of the International Narcotics Control Board (www.incb.org).

TABLE DES MATIÈRES

*Les annexes ne figurent ni dans la version imprimée ni dans la version électronique de la présente publication, mais sont disponibles sur le site Web de l'Organe international de contrôle des stupéfiants (www.incb.org).

ÍNDICE

*Los anexos no se incluyen ni en la versión impresa ni en la versión electrónica de la presente publicación, pero pueden consultarse en el sitio web de la Junta Internacional de Fiscalización de Estupefacientes (www.incb.org).

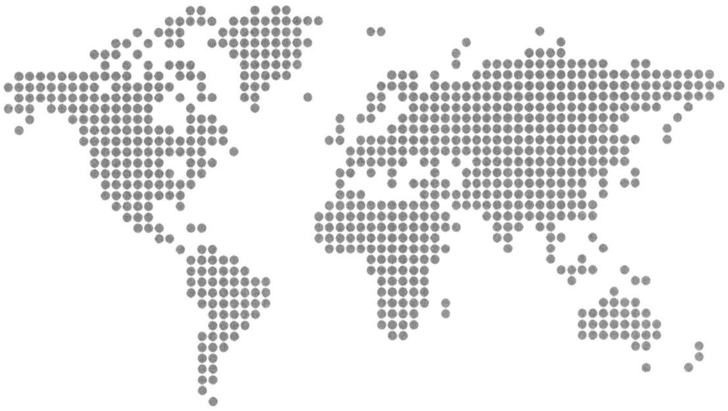

Part one
Première partie
Primera parte

Introduction

1. In addition to its annual report, the International Narcotics Control Board (INCB) publishes technical information in accordance with the following provisions of the Convention on Psychotropic Substances of 1971:

Article 18. Reports of the Board

> 1. The Board shall prepare annual reports on its work containing an analysis of the statistical information at its disposal, and, in appropriate cases, an account of the explanations, if any, given by or required of Governments, together with any observations and recommendations which the Board desires to make. The Board may make such additional reports as it considers necessary. The reports shall be submitted to the Council through the Commission, which may make such comments as it sees fit.
>
> 2. The reports of the Board shall be communicated to the Parties and subsequently published by the Secretary-General. The Parties shall permit their unrestricted distribution.

2. The technical data are published for control purposes and to meet the needs of researchers, enterprises and the general public. Pursuant to the provisions of article 16, paragraph 4, parties are required to furnish to the Board annual statistical reports relating to the substances listed in Schedules I–IV of the 1971 Convention. The statistical data that parties to the 1971 Convention are required to furnish to the Board differ according to the Schedule in which a given substance is included. The individual tables of the present technical report are based on those data.

3. Data reported later than 1 November 2024 could not be taken into consideration in preparing this technical report.

Introduction

1. Outre son rapport annuel, l'Organe international de contrôle des stupéfiants (OICS) publie des informations techniques conformément aux dispositions ci-après de la Convention sur les substances psychotropes de 1971.

Article 18. Rapports de l'Organe

> 1. L'Organe établit sur ses travaux des rapports annuels dans lesquels figurent une analyse des renseignements statistiques dont il dispose et, dans les cas appropriés, un exposé des explications que les gouvernements ont pu fournir ou ont été requis de fournir, ainsi que toute observation et recommandation que l'Organe peut vouloir formuler. L'Organe peut également faire tous rapports supplémentaires qu'il peut juger nécessaires. Les rapports sont présentés au Conseil par l'intermédiaire de la Commission qui peut formuler les observations qu'elle juge opportunes.
>
> 2. Les rapports de l'Organe sont communiqués aux Parties et publiés ultérieurement par le Secrétaire général. Les Parties autorisent la libre distribution de ces rapports.

2. Les renseignements techniques sont publiés à des fins de contrôle et à l'intention des chercheurs, des entreprises et du public. Conformément aux dispositions du paragraphe 4 de l'article 16, les Parties sont tenues de fournir à l'OICS des rapports statistiques annuels sur les substances des Tableaux I à IV de la Convention de 1971. Les informations statistiques que les Parties à la Convention de 1971 ont l'obligation de fournir à l'OICS varient selon le Tableau auquel appartient une substance donnée. Les différents tableaux du présent rapport technique sont basés sur ces données.

3. Les données communiquées après le 1er novembre 2024 n'ont pas été prises en compte pour la préparation du présent rapport technique.

Introducción

1. La Junta Internacional de Fiscalización de Estupefacientes (JIFE) publica, además de su informe anual, información técnica de conformidad con las siguientes disposiciones del Convenio sobre Sustancias Sicotrópicas de 1971:

Artículo 18. Informes de la Junta

> 1. La Junta preparará informes anuales sobre su labor; dichos informes contendrán un análisis de los datos estadísticos de que disponga la Junta y, cuando proceda, una reseña de las declaraciones hechas por los gobiernos o que se les hayan pedido, si las hubiere, junto con las observaciones y recomendaciones que la Junta desee hacer. La Junta podrá preparar los informes complementarios que considere necesarios. Los informes serán sometidos al Consejo por intermedio de la Comisión, que formulará las observaciones que estime oportunas.
>
> 2. Los informes de la Junta serán comunicados a las Partes y publicados posteriormente por el Secretario General. Las Partes permitirán que se distribuyan sin restricciones.

2. Los datos técnicos se publican para fines de control y para satisfacer las necesidades de los investigadores, las empresas y el público en general. En cumplimiento de lo dispuesto en el párrafo 4 del artículo 16, se pide a las partes que faciliten a la Junta informes estadísticos anuales en relación con las sustancias incluidas en las Listas I a IV del Convenio de 1971. Los datos estadísticos que las partes en el Convenio de 1971 deben suministrar a la Junta varían según la Lista en la cual esté incluida la sustancia de que se trate. En los diferentes cuadros del presente informe técnico se resumen esos datos.

3. Los datos comunicados después del 1.° de noviembre de 2024 no se pudieron tener en cuenta al preparar este informe técnico.

Table I. Parties and non-parties to the Convention on Psychotropic Substances of 1971, by region

Tableau I. Parties et non-parties à la Convention sur les substances psychotropes de 1971, par région

Cuadro I. Partes y no partes en el Convenio sobre Sustancias Sicotrópicas de 1971, por región

Region Région Región	Party to the 1971 Convention[a] Partie à la Convention de 1971[a] Parte en el Convenio de 1971[a]		Non-party to the 1971 Convention Non-partie à la Convention de 1971 No parte en el Convenio de 1971
Africa **Afrique** **África** *Number of States:* *Nombre d'États:* *Número de Estados:* 54 *Parties:* *Parties:* *Partes:* 51 *Non-parties:* *Non-parties:* *No partes:* 3	Algeria (14.7.1978) Algérie Argelia Angola (26.10.2005) Benin (6.11.1973) Bénin Botswana (27.12.1984) Burkina Faso (20.1.1987) Burundi (18.2.1993) Cameroon (5.6.1981) Cameroun Camerún Cabo Verde (24.5.1990) Central African Rep. (15.10.2001) République centrafricaine República Centroafricana Chad (9.6.1995) Tchad Comoros (1.3.2000) Comores Comoras Congo (3.3.2004) Côte d'Ivoire (11.4.1984)	Dem. Rep. of the Congo (12.10.1977) Rép. dém. du Congo Rep. Dem. del Congo Djibouti (22.2.2001) Egypt (14.6.1972) Égypte Egipto Eritrea (30.1.2002) Erythrée Eswatini (3.10.1995) Ethiopia (23.6.1980) Éthiopie Etiopía Gabon (14.10.1981) Gabón Gambia (23.4.1996) Gambie Ghana (10.4.1990) Guinea (27.12.1990) Guinée Guinea-Bissau (27.10.1995) Guinée-Bissau Kenya (18.10.2000)	Equatorial Guinea Guinée équatoriale Guinea Ecuatorial Liberia Libéria South Sudan Soudan du Sud Sudán del Sur

Table I. Parties and non-parties to the 1971 Convention *(continued)*
Tableau I. Parties et non-parties à la Convention de 1971 *(suite)*
Cuadro I. Partes y no partes en el Convenio de 1971 *(continuación)*

Region Région Región	Party to the 1971 Convention[a] Partie à la Convention de 1971[a] Parte en el Convenio de 1971[a]	Non-party to the 1971 Convention Non-partie à la Convention de 1971 No parte en el Convenio de 1971
Africa Afrique África	Lesotho (23.4.1975)	
	Libya (24.4.1979) Libye Libia	
	Madagascar (20.6.1974)	
	Malawi (9.4.1980)	
	Mali (31.10.95) Malí	
	Mauritania (24.10.1989) Mauritanie	
	Mauritius (8.5.1973) Maurice Mauricio	
	Morocco (11.2.1980) Maroc Marruecos	
	Mozambique (8.6.1998)	
	Namibia (31.3.1998) Namibie	
	Niger (10.11.1992) Níger	
	Nigeria (23.6.1981) Nigéria	
	Rwanda (15.7.1981)	
	Sao Tome and Principe (20.6.1996) Sao Tomé-et-Principe Santo Tomé y Príncipe	
	Senegal (10.6.1977) Sénégal	
	Seychelles (27.2.1992)	
	Sierra Leone (6.6.1994) Sierra Leona	
	Somalia (2.9.1986) Somalie	
	South Africa (27.1.1972) Afrique du Sud Sudáfrica	
	Sudan (26.7.1993) Soudan Sudán	
	Togo (18.5.1976)	
	Tunisia (23.7.1979) Tunisie Túnez	
	Uganda (15.4.1988) Ouganda	
	United Republic of Tanzania (7.12.2000) République-Unie de Tanzanie República Unida de Tanzanía	
	Zambia (28.5.1993) Zambie	
	Zimbabwe (30.7.1993)	

Table I. Parties and non-parties to the 1971 Convention *(continued)*
Tableau I. Parties et non-parties à la Convention de 1971 *(suite)*
Cuadro I. Partes y no partes en el Convenio de 1971 *(continuación)*

Region Région Región	Party to the 1971 Convention[a] Partie à la Convention de 1971[a] Parte en el Convenio de 1971[a]	Non-party to the 1971 Convention Non-partie à la Convention de 1971 No parte en el Convenio de 1971
The Americas **Les Amériques** **Las Américas** *Number of States:* *Nombre d'États:* *Número de Estados:* 35 *Parties:* *Parties:* *Partes:* 34 *Non-parties:* *Non-parties:* *No partes:* 1	Antigua and Barbuda (5.4.1993) Antigua-et-Barbuda Antigua y Barbuda Argentina (16.2.1978) Argentine Bahamas (31.8.1987) Barbados (28.1.1975) Barbade Belize (18.12.2001) Belice Bolivia (Plurinational State of) (20.3.1985) Bolivie (État plurinational de) Bolivia (Estado Pluri-nacional de) Brazil (14.2.1973) Brésil Brasil Canada (10.9.1988) Canadá Chile (18.5.1972) Chili Colombia (12.5.1981) Colombie Costa Rica (16.2.1977) Cuba (26.4.1976) Dominica (24.9.1993) Dominique Dominican Republic (19.11.1975) République dominicaine República Dominicana Ecuador (7.9.1973) Équateur El Salvador (11.6.1998) Grenada (25.4.1980) Grenade Granada Guatemala (13.8.1979) Guyana (4.5.1977) Honduras (23.5.2005) Jamaica (6.10.1989) Jamaïque Mexico (20.2.1975) Mexique México Nicaragua (24.10.1973) Panama (18.2.1972) Panamá Paraguay (3.2.1972) Peru (28.1.1980) Pérou Perú Saint Kitts and Nevis (9.5.1994) Saint-Kitts-et-Névis Saint Kitts y Nevis Saint Lucia (16.1.2003) Sainte-Lucie Santa Lucía Saint Vincent and the Grenadines (3.12.2001) Saint-Vincent-et-les Grenadines San Vicente y las Granadinas Suriname (29.3.1990) Trinidad and Tobago (14.3.1979) Trinité-et-Tobago Trinidad y Tabago United States (16.4.1980) États-Unis Estados Unidos Uruguay (16.3.1976) Venezuela (Bolivarian Rep. of) (23.5.1972) Venezuela (Rép. bolivarienne du) Venezuela (Rep. Bolivariana de)	Haiti Haïti Haití

Table I. Parties and non-parties to the 1971 Convention *(continued)*
Tableau I. Parties et non-parties à la Convention de 1971 *(suite)*
Cuadro I. Partes y no partes en el Convenio de 1971 *(continuación)*

Region Région Región	Party to the 1971 Convention[a] Partie à la Convention de 1971[a] Parte en el Convenio de 1971[a]	Non-party to the 1971 Convention Non-partie à la Convention de 1971 No parte en el Convenio de 1971
Asia **Asie** *Number of States:* *Nombre d'États:* *Número de Estados:* 47 Parties: Parties: Partes: 46 *Non-parties:* *Non-parties:* *No partes:* 1	Afghanistan (21.5.1985) Afganistán Armenia (13.9.1993) Arménie Azerbaijan (11.1.1999) Azerbaïdjan Azerbaiyán Bahrain (7.2.1990) Bahreïn Bahrein Bangladesh (11.10.1990) Bhutan (18.8.2005) Bhoutan Bhután Brunei Darussalam (24.11.1987) Brunéi Darussalam Cambodia (7.7.2005) Cambodge Camboya China (23.8.1985) Chine Democratic People's Republic of Korea (19.3.2007) République populaire démocratique de Corée República Popular Democrática de Corea Georgia (8.1.1998) Géorgie India (23.4.1975) Inde Indonesia (19.12.1996) Indonésie Iran (Islamic Rep. of) (9.8.2000) Iran (Rép. islamique d') Irán (Rep. Islámica del) Iraq (17.5.1976) Israel (10.6.1993) Israël Japan (31.8.1990) Japon Japón Jordan (8.8.1975) Jordanie Jordania Kazakhstan (29.4.1997) Kazajstán Kuwait (13.7.1979) Koweït Kyrgyzstan (7.10.1994) Kirghizistan Kirguistán Lao People's Democratic Republic (22.9.1997) République démocratique populaire lao República Democrática Popular Lao Lebanon (15.12.1994) Liban Líbano Malaysia (22.7.1986) Malaisie Malasia Maldives (7.9.2000) Maldivas Mongolia (15.12.1999) Mongolie Myanmar (21.9.1995) Nepal (9.2.2007) Népal Oman (3.7.1997) Omán	Timor-Leste

Table I. Parties and non-parties to the 1971 Convention *(continued)*
Tableau I. Parties et non-parties à la Convention de 1971 *(suite)*
Cuadro I. Partes y no partes en el Convenio de 1971 *(continuación)*

Region Région Región	Party to the 1971 Convention[a] Partie à la Convention de 1971[a] Parte en el Convenio de 1971[a]		Non-party to the 1971 Convention Non-partie à la Convention de 1971 No parte en el Convenio de 1971
Asia **Asie**	Pakistan (9.6.1977) Pakistán Philippines (7.6.1974) Filipinas Qatar (18.12.1986) Rep. of Korea (12.1.1978) République de Corée República de Corea Saudi Arabia (29.1.1975) Arabie saoudite Arabia Saudita Singapore (17.9.1990) Singapour Singapur Sri Lanka (15.3.1993) State of Palestine (29.12.2017) État de Palestine Estado de Palestina Syrian Arab Rep. (8.3.1976) République arabe syrienne República Árabe Siria	Tajikistan (26.3.1997) Tadjikistan Tayikistán Thailand (21.11.1975) Thaïlande Tailandia Türkiye (1.4.1981) Turkmenistan (21.2.1996) Turkménistan Turkmenistán United Arab Emirates (17.2.1988) Émirats arabes unis Emiratos Árabes Unidos Uzbekistan (12.7.1995) Ouzbékistan Uzbekistán Viet Nam (4.11.1997) Yemen (25.3.1996) Yémen	
Europe **Europa** *Number of States:* *Nombre d'États:* *Número de Estados:* 45 *Parties:* *Parties:* *Partes:* 45 *Non-parties:* *Non-parties:* *No partes:* 0	Albania (24.1.2003) Albanie Andorra (13.2.2007) Andorre Austria (23.6.1997) Autriche Belarus (15.12.1978) Bélarus Belarús Belgium (25.10.1995) Belgique Bélgica Bosnia and Herzegovina (1.9.1993) Bosnie-Herzégovine Bosnia y Herzegovina	Bulgaria (18.5.1972) Bulgarie Croatia (26.7.1993) Croatie Croacia Cyprus (26.11.1973) Chypre Chipre Czechia (30.12.1993) Tchéquie Chequia Denmark (18.4.1975) Danemark Dinamarca	

Table I. Parties and non-parties to the 1971 Convention *(continued)*
Tableau I. Parties et non-parties à la Convention de 1971 *(suite)*
Cuadro I. Partes y no partes en el Convenio de 1971 *(continuación)*

Region Région Región	Party to the 1971 Convention[a] Partie à la Convention de 1971[a] Parte en el Convenio de 1971[a]		Non-party to the 1971 Convention Non-partie à la Convention de 1971 No parte en el Convenio de 1971
Europe **Europa**	Estonia (5.7.1996) Estonie Finland (20.11.1972) Finlande Finlandia France (28.1.1975) Francia Germany (2.12.1977) Allemagne Alemania Greece (10.2.1977) Grèce Grecia Holy See (7.1.1976) Saint-Siège Santa Sede Hungary (19.7.1979) Hongrie Hungría Iceland (18.12.1974) Islande Islandia Ireland (7.8.1992) Irlande Irlanda Italy (27.11.1981) Italie Italia Latvia (16.7.1993) Lettonie Letonia Liechtenstein (24.11.1999) Lithuania (28.2.1994) Lituanie Lituania	Luxembourg (7.2.1991) Luxemburgo Malta (22.2.1990) Malte Monaco (6.7.1977) Mónaco Montenegro (23.10.2006) Monténégro Netherlands (Kingdom of the) (8.9.1993) Pays-Bas (Royaume des) Países Bajos (Reino de los) North Macedonia (13.10.1993) Macédoine du Nord Macedonia del Norte Norway (18.7.1975) Norvège Noruega Poland (3.1.1975) Pologne Polonia Portugal (20.4.1979) Rep. of Moldova (15.2.1995) Rép. de Moldova Rep. de Moldova Romania (21.1.1993) Roumanie Rumania Russian Federation (3.11.1978) Fédération de Russie Federación de Rusia San Marino (10.10.2000) Saint-Marin Serbia (12.3.2001) Serbie	

Table I. Parties and non-parties to the 1971 Convention *(continued)*
Tableau I. Parties et non-parties à la Convention de 1971 *(suite)*
Cuadro I. Partes y no partes en el Convenio de 1971 *(continuación)*

Region Région Región	Party to the 1971 Convention[a] Partie à la Convention de 1971[a] Parte en el Convenio de 1971[a]		Non-party to the 1971 Convention Non-partie à la Convention de 1971 No parte en el Convenio de 1971	
Europe **Europa**	Slovakia (28.5.1993) Slovaquie Eslovaquia Slovenia (6.7.1992) Slovénie Eslovenia Spain (20.7.1973) Espagne España Sweden (5.12.1972) Suède Suecia	Switzerland (22.4.1996) Suisse Suiza Ukraine (20.11.1978) Ucrania United Kingdom (24.3.1986) Royaume-Uni Reino Unido		
Oceania **Océanie** **Oceanía** *Number of States:* *Nombre d'États:* *Número de Estados:* 16 *Parties:* *Parties:* *Partes:* 8 *Non-parties:* *Non-parties:* *No partes:* 8	Australia (19.5.1982) Australie Fiji (25.3.1993) Fidji Marshall Islands (9.8.1991) Îles Marshall Islas Marshall Micronesia (Federated States of) (29.4.1991) Micronésie (États fédérés de) Micronesia (Estados Federados de)	New Zealand (7.6.1990) Nouvelle-Zélande Nueva Zelandia Palau (19.8.1998) Palaos Papua New Guinea (20.11.1981) Papouasie-Nouvelle-Guinée Papua Nueva Guinea Tonga (24.10.1975)	Cook Islands Îles Cook Islas Cook Kiribati Nauru Niue Nioué Samoa Solomon Islands Îles Salomon Islas Salomón Tuvalu	Vanuatu

World total	*Number of States — Nombre d'États — Número de Estados*	197
Total mondial	*Parties — Parties — Partes*	184
Total mundial	*Non-parties — Non-parties — No partes*	13

[a]For parties, the dates on which the instruments of ratification or accession were deposited are indicated in parentheses. — Pour les parties, la date du dépôt des instruments de ratification ou d'adhésion est indiquée entre parenthèses. — Para los países que son partes en el Convenio, se indican entre paréntesis las fechas en que se depositaron los instrumentos de ratificación o adhesión.

Table II. Receipt of statistics for 2023

Table II reflects the extent of compliance by Governments with the provisions of article 16 of the 1971 Convention in submitting to INCB annual statistical information for 2023. The table also shows to what extent Governments have voluntarily submitted additional information to INCB, pursuant to recommendations of the Board endorsed by the Economic and Social Council and by the Commission on Narcotic Drugs, that is, quarterly statistics on international trade in substances in Schedule II (Council resolution 1981/7) and statistics on the consumption of psychotropic substances (Commission resolution 54/6). The following symbols are used in table II:

A dash (—) indicates that the statistical report for 2023 had not been received by 1 November 2024;

The symbol "×" indicates that the competent administration has furnished for 2023 at least part of the required statistical information;

Countries and non-metropolitan territories are listed in English alphabetical order; the names of territories are shown in italics. The names of countries and territories are those that were in official use at the time the data were collected (in 2023).

Tableau II. Réception des statistiques pour 2023

Le tableau II indique quels gouvernements se sont conformés aux dispositions de l'article 16 de la Convention de 1971 en soumettant à l'OICS des statistiques annuelles pour 2023. Ce tableau indique aussi dans quelle mesure les gouvernements ont volontairement soumis à l'OICS des informations supplémentaires, conformément aux recommandations de l'OICS approuvées par le Conseil économique et social et par la Commission des stupéfiants, c'est-à-dire des statistiques trimestrielles sur le commerce international des substances du Tableau II (résolution 1981/7 du Conseil) et des statistiques sur la consommation de substances psychotropes (résolution 54/6 de la Commission). Dans ce tableau, les symboles suivants ont été utilisés:

Un tiret (—) indique que le rapport statistique pour 2023 n'avait pas été reçu au 1er novembre 2024;

Le signe "×" indique que l'administration compétente a fourni au moins une partie des données statistiques requises pour 2023;

Les pays et territoires figurent dans l'ordre alphabétique anglais; les noms des territoires apparaissent en italique. Les noms des pays et territoires sont ceux qui étaient officiellement en usage au moment où les données ont été recueillies (en 2023).

Cuadro II. Recepción de las estadísticas de 2023

En el cuadro II se refleja la medida en que los gobiernos cumplen con las disposiciones del artículo 16 del Convenio de 1971 en lo que respecta a la presentación a la JIFE de la información estadística anual correspondiente a 2023. En el cuadro también se indica en qué medida los gobiernos han presentado voluntariamente a la JIFE, en cumplimiento de las recomendaciones de la Junta, que hicieron suyas el Consejo Económico y Social y la Comisión de Estupefacientes, información adicional, como estadísticas trimestrales sobre comercio internacional de sustancias incluidas en la Lista II (resolución 1981/7 del Consejo Económico y Social) y estadísticas sobre el consumo de sustancias sicotrópicas (resolución 54/6 de la Comisión). En dicho cuadro se utilizan los símbolos siguientes:

La raya (—) indica que al 1 de noviembre de 2024 no se había recibido el informe estadístico correspondiente a 2023;

El signo "×" indica que la administración competente ha facilitado por lo menos una parte de la información estadística requerida correspondiente a 2023;

Los países y territorios no metropolitanos se enumeran en orden alfabético inglés; los nombres de los territorios aparecen en letra cursiva. Los nombres de los países y territorios son los que se utilizaban oficialmente en el momento en que se obtuvo la información (en 2023).

Table II. Receipt of statistics for 2023
Tableau II. Réception des statistiques pour 2023
Cuadro II. Recepción de las estadísticas de 2023

Country or territory Pays ou territoire País o territorio	Annual statistics Statistiques annuelles Estadísticas anuales	Quarterly statistics Statistiques trimestrielles Estadísticas trimestrales Schedule II Tableau II Lista II				Reported consumption[a] La consommation déclarée[a] Consumo declarado[a]
		Q1	Q2	Q3	Q4	
Afghanistan — Afganistán	—	—	—	—	—	—
Albania — Albanie	×	×	×	×	×	×
Algeria — Algérie — Argelia	×	—	—	—	—	—
Andorra — Andorre	×	×	×	×	×	—
Angola	×	—	×	×	×	×
Anguilla — Anguila	—	—	—	—	—	—
Antigua and Barbuda — Antigua-et-Barbuda — Antigua y Barbuda	—	—	—	—	—	—
Argentina — Argentine	×	—	—	—	—	—
Armenia — Arménie	×	—	—	—	—	×
Aruba	—	—	—	—	—	—
Ascension — Isla de la Ascensión	×	—	—	—	—	×
Australia — Australie	×	×	×	×	×	×
Austria — Autriche	×	×	×	×	×	×
Azerbaijan — Azerbaïdjan — Azerbaiyán	×	×	×	×	×	—
Bahamas	—	—	—	—	—	—
Bahrain — Bahreïn — Bahrein	×	×	×	×	×	×
Bangladesh	×	—	—	—	—	—
Barbados — Barbade	×	×	×	×	×	—
Belarus — Bélarus — Belarús	×	×	×	×	×	×
Belgium — Belgique — Bélgica	×	×	×	×	×	×
Belize — Belice	×	—	—	—	—	×
Benin — Bénin	—	—	—	—	—	—
Bermuda — Bermudes — Bermudas	—	—	—	—	—	—
Bhutan — Bhoutan — Bhután	×	—	—	—	—	×
Bolivia (Plurinational State of) — Bolivie (État plurinational de) — Bolivia (Estado Plurinacional de)	×	×	×	×	×	×
Bosnia and Herzegovina — Bosnie-Herzégovine — Bosnia y Herzegovina	×	—	—	—	—	×
Botswana	×	×	×	×	×	—
Brazil — Brésil — Brasil	×	×	×	×	—	×

Table II. Receipt of statistics for 2023 *(continued)*
Tableau II. Réception des statistiques pour 2023 *(suite)*
Cuadro II. Recepción de las estadísticas de 2023 *(continuación)*

Country or territory / Pays ou territoire / País o territorio	Annual statistics / Statistiques annuelles / Estadísticas anuales	Quarterly statistics / Statistiques trimestrielles / Estadísticas trimestrales — Schedule II / Tableau II / Lista II				Reported consumption[a] / La consommation déclarée[a] / Consumo declarado[a]
		Q1	Q2	Q3	Q4	
British Virgin Islands — Îles Vierges britanniques — Islas Vírgenes Británicas	—	×	—	—	—	—
Brunei Darussalam — Brunéi Darussalam	×	×	×	×	×	—
Bulgaria — Bulgarie	×	×	×	×	×	×
Burkina Faso	×	—	—	—	—	×
Burundi	×	—	—	—	—	×
Cabo Verde	×	×	×	×	×	×
Cambodia — Cambodge — Camboya	—	—	—	—	—	—
Cameroon — Cameroun — Camerún	×	×	×	×	×	—
Canada — Canadá	×	×	×	×	×	×
Cayman Islands — Îles Caïmanes — Islas Caiman	—	—	—	—	—	—
Central African Republic — République centrafricaine — República Centroafricana	—	—	—	—	—	—
Chad — Tchad	×	—	—	—	—	—
Chile — Chili	×	×	—	×	×	×
China — Chine	×	×	×	×	×	×
China, Hong Kong SAR — Chine, RAS de Hong Kong — China, RAE de Hong Kong	×	×	×	×	×	—
China, Macao SAR — Chine, RAS de Macao — China, RAE de Macao	×	×	—	×	×	×
Christmas Island — Île Christmas — Isla Christmas	×	×	×	×	×	—
Cocos (Keeling) Islands	×	×	×	×	×	—
Colombia — Colombie	×	×	×	×	×	×
Comoros — Comores — Comoras	×	—	—	—	—	×
Congo	—	—	—	—	—	—
Cook Islands[b] — Îles Cook[b] — Islas Cook[b]	×	—	—	—	—	—
Costa Rica	×	×	×	×	×	×
Côte d'Ivoire	×	—	×	×	×	—
Croatia — Croatie — Croacia	×	×	×	×	×	—
Cuba	×	—	—	×	×	×

Table II. Receipt of statistics for 2023 *(continued)*
Tableau II. Réception des statistiques pour 2023 *(suite)*
Cuadro II. Recepción de las estadísticas de 2023 *(continuación)*

Country or territory Pays ou territoire País o territorio	Annual statistics Statistiques annuelles Estadísticas anuales	Quarterly statistics Statistiques trimestrielles Estadísticas trimestrales Schedule II Tableau II Lista II				Reported consumption[a] La consommation déclarée[a] Consumo declarado[a]
		Q1	Q2	Q3	Q4	
Curaçao	×	×	×	—	—	—
Cyprus — Chypre — Chipre	×	×	×	×	×	—
Czechia — Tchéquie — Chequia	×	×	×	×	×	×
Dem. People's Republic of Korea — République populaire dém. de Corée — República Popular Dem. de Corea	×	—	—	—	—	—
Democratic Republic of the Congo — République démocratique du Congo — República Democrática del Congo	×	×	—	—	—	—
Denmark — Danemark — Dinamarca	×	×	×	×	×	×
Djibouti	—	—	—	—	—	—
Dominica — Dominique	—	—	—	—	—	—
Dominican Republic — République dominicaine — República Dominicana	×	×	—	×	×	×
Ecuador — Équateur	×	×	×	×	×	×
Egypt — Égypte — Egipto	×	×	×	×	×	—
El Salvador	×	×	×	×	×	×
Equatorial Guinea[b] — Guinée équatoriale[b] — Guinea Ecuatorial[b]	—	—	—	—	—	—
Eritrea — Érythrée	×	—	—	—	—	×
Estonia — Estonie	×	×	×	×	×	×
Eswatini	×	—	—	—	—	—
Ethiopia — Éthiopie — Etiopía	×	—	—	—	—	—
Falkland Islands (Malvinas) — Îles Falkland (Malvinas) — Islas Malvinas (Falkland Islands)	×	×	×	×	×	×
Fiji — Fidji	×	—	—	—	—	—
Finland — Finlande — Finlandia	×	×	×	×	×	×
France — Francia	×	—	—	—	—	×
French Polynesia — Polynésie française — Polinesia Francesa	×	—	—	—	—	—
Gabon — Gabón	×	—	×	—	—	—
Gambia — Gambie	—	—	—	—	—	—
Georgia — Géorgie	×	×	×	×	×	×
Germany — Allemagne — Alemania	×	×	×	×	×	×

Table II. Receipt of statistics for 2023 *(continued)*
Tableau II. Réception des statistiques pour 2023 *(suite)*
Cuadro II. Recepción de las estadísticas de 2023 *(continuación)*

Country or territory Pays ou territoire País o territorio	Annual statistics Statistiques annuelles Estadísticas anuales	Quarterly statistics / Statistiques trimestrielles / Estadísticas trimestrales Schedule II / Tableau II / Lista II				Reported consumption[a] La consommation déclarée[a] Consumo declarado[a]
		Q1	Q2	Q3	Q4	
Ghana	×	×	×	×	×	—
Gibraltar	×	×	×	×	×	×
Greece — Grèce — Grecia	×	×	×	×	×	×
Grenada — Grenade — Granada	×	—	—	×	—	×
Guatemala	×	×	×	×	×	×
Guinea — Guinée	×	—	—	—	—	×
Guinea-Bissau — Guinée-Bissau	—	—	—	—	—	—
Guyana	×	×	×	×	×	×
Haiti[b] — Haïti[b] — Haití[b]	×	×	×	×	×	—
Holy See[c] — Saint-Siège[c] — Santa Sede[c]	—	—	—	—	—	—
Honduras	×	×	×	×	×	—
Hungary — Hongrie — Hungría	×	×	×	×	×	×
Iceland — Islande — Islandia	×	×	×	×	×	×
India — Inde	×	×	×	×	×	×
Indonesia — Indonésie	×	×	×	×	×	—
Iran (Islamic Republic of) — Iran (République islamique d') — Irán (República Islámica del)	—	×	×	×	×	—
Iraq	×	×	×	×	—	×
Ireland — Irlande — Irlanda	×	×	×	×	×	—
Israel — Israël	×	×	×	×	×	×
Italy — Italie — Italia	×	×	×	×	×	×
Jamaica — Jamaïque	×	×	×	×	×	×
Japan — Japon — Japón	×	×	×	×	×	—
Jordan — Jordanie — Jordania	×	×	×	×	×	—
Kazakhstan — Kazajstán	×	—	—	—	—	—
Kenya	×	×	—	—	×	×
Kiribati[b]	—	—	—	—	—	—
Kuwait — Koweït	×	×	×	×	×	—
Kyrgyzstan — Kirghizistan — Kirguistán	×	×	×	×	×	×
Lao People's Democratic Rep. — Rép. démocratique populaire lao — Rep. Democrática Popular Lao	—	×	×	×	×	—
Latvia — Lettonie — Letonia	×	×	×	×	×	×
Lebanon — Liban — Líbano	×	×	×	×	×	×

Table II. Receipt of statistics for 2023 *(continued)*
Tableau II. Réception des statistiques pour 2023 *(suite)*
Cuadro II. Recepción de las estadísticas de 2023 *(continuación)*

Country or territory Pays ou territoire País o territorio	Annual statistics Statistiques annuelles Estadísticas anuales	Quarterly statistics Statistiques trimestrielles Estadísticas trimestrales Schedule II Tableau II Lista II				Reported consumption[a] La consommation déclarée[a] Consumo declarado[a]
		Q1	Q2	Q3	Q4	
Lesotho	—	—	—	—	—	—
Liberia[b] — Libéria[b]	×	×	×	×	×	×
Libya — Libie — Libia	—	—	—	—	—	—
Liechtenstein[d]	—	—	—	—	—	—
Lithuania — Lituanie — Lituania	×	×	×	×	×	×
Luxembourg — Luxemburgo	×	×	×	×	×	×
Madagascar	×	×	×	—	—	×
Malawi	×	—	—	—	—	×
Malaysia — Malaisie — Malasia	×	×	×	×	×	×
Maldives — Maldivas	×	×	×	×	×	×
Mali — Malí	—	—	—	—	—	—
Malta — Malte	×	×	×	×	×	×
Marshall Islands — Îles Marshall — Islas Marshall	×		—	—	—	×
Mauritania — Mauritanie	×	—	—	—	—	×
Mauritius — Maurice — Mauricio	×	—	—	—	—	—
Mexico — Mexique — México	×	—	—	×	—	×
Micronesia (Federated States of) — Micronésie (États fédérés de) — Micronesia (Estados Federados de)	×	—	—	—	—	×
Monaco[e] — Mónaco[e]	—	—	—	—	—	—
Mongolia — Mongolie	×	×	×	×	×	—
Montenegro — Monténégro	×	×	×	×	×	×
Montserrat	×	×	×	×	×	—
Morocco — Maroc — Marruecos	×	×	×	×	×	×
Mozambique	×	×	×	×	×	×
Myanmar	×	×	×	×	×	—
Namibia — Namibie	×	×	×	×	×	—
Nauru[b]	—	—	—	—	—	—
Nepal — Népal	×	—	—	—	—	—
Netherlands (Kingdom of the) — Pays-Bas (Royaume des) — Países Bajos (Reino de los)	×	×	×	—	×	×
New Caledonia — Nouvelle-Calédonie — Nueva Caledonia	—	×	×	×	×	—

Table II. Receipt of statistics for 2023 *(continued)*
Tableau II. Réception des statistiques pour 2023 *(suite)*
Cuadro II. Recepción de las estadísticas de 2023 *(continuación)*

Country or territory Pays ou territoire País o territorio	Annual statistics Statistiques annuelles Estadísticas anuales	Quarterly statistics Statistiques trimestrielles Estadísticas trimestrales				Reported consumption[a] La consommation déclarée[a] Consumo declarado[a]
		Schedule II Tableau II Lista II				
		Q1	Q2	Q3	Q4	
New Zealand — Nouvelle-Zélande — Nueva Zelandia	×	×	×	×	×	×
Nicaragua	×	×	×	×	×	—
Niger — Níger	—	—	—	—	—	—
Nigeria — Nigéria	×	×	×	×	—	—
Niue[b] — Nioué[b]	×	—	—	—	—	×
Norfolk Island — Île Norfolk — Isla Norfolk	×	×	×	×	×	—
North Macedonia — Macédoine du Nord — Macedonia del Norte	×	—	×	×	×	×
Norway — Norvège — Noruega	×	×	×	×	×	×
Oman — Omán	×	×	×	×	×	—
Pakistan — Pakistán	×	×	×	×	—	—
Palau — Palaos	×	×	×	×	×	×
Panama — Panamá	×	×	×	×	×	—
Papua New Guinea — Papouasie-Nouvelle-Guinée — Papua Nueva Guinea	—	—	—	—	—	—
Paraguay	×	×	×	×	×	—
Peru — Pérou — Perú	×	×	×	×	×	×
Philippines — Filipinas	×	×	×	×	×	—
Poland — Pologne — Polonia	×	—	—	—	×	×
Portugal	×	×	×	×	×	×
Qatar	×	×	×	×	×	×
Republic of Korea — République de Corée — República de Corea	×	—	×	×	×	×
Republic of Moldova — République de Moldova — República de Moldova	—	—	—	—	—	—
Romania — Roumanie — Rumania	×	×	×	×	×	×
Russian Federation — Fédération de Russie — Federación de Rusia	×	×	×	×	×	—
Rwanda	×	—	—	—	—	—
Saint Helena — Sainte-Hélène — Santa Elena	×	—	—	—	—	×

Table II. Receipt of statistics for 2023 *(continued)*
Tableau II. Réception des statistiques pour 2023 *(suite)*
Cuadro II. Recepción de las estadísticas de 2023 *(continuación)*

Country or territory Pays ou territoire País o territorio	Annual statistics Statistiques annuelles Estadísticas anuales	Quarterly statistics / Statistiques trimestrielles / Estadísticas trimestrales Schedule II / Tableau II / Lista II				Reported consumption[a] La consommation déclarée[a] Consumo declarado[a]
		Q1	Q2	Q3	Q4	
Saint Kitts and Nevis — Saint-Kitts-et-Nevis — Saint Kitts y Nevis	×	—	—	—	—	—
Saint Lucia — Sainte-Lucie — Santa Lucía	×	×	—	—	—	—
Saint Vincent and the Grenadines — Saint-Vincent-et-les Grenadines — San Vicente y las Granadinas	×	×	×	×	×	×
Samoa[b]	—	—	—	—	—	—
San Marino — Saint-Marin	×	—	—	—	—	×
Sao Tome and Principe — Sao Tomé-et-Principe — Santo Tomé y Príncipe	—	—	—	—	—	—
Saudi Arabia — Arabie saoudite — Arabia Saudita	×	×	×	×	×	—
Senegal — Sénégal	×	—	—	—	—	—
Serbia — Serbie	×	×	×	×	×	—
Seychelles	×	×	×	×	×	×
Sierra Leone — Sierra Leona	×	×	×	×	×	×
Singapore — Singapour — Singapur	×	×	×	×	×	×
Sint Maarten — Saint-Martin — San Martín	×	×	×	×	×	×
Slovakia — Slovaquie — Eslovaquia	×	×	×	×	—	—
Slovenia — Slovénie — Eslovenia	×	×	×	×	×	×
Solomon Islands[b] — Îles Salomon[b] — Islas Salomón[b]	×	—	—	—	—	×
Somalia — Somalie	×	—	—	—	—	×
South Africa — Afrique du Sud — Sudáfrica	×	—	—	—	—	×
South Sudan[b] — Soudan du Sud[b] — Sudán del Sur[b]	—	—	—	—	—	—
Spain — Espagne — España	×	×	×	×	×	×
Sri Lanka	×	×	×	×	×	×
Sudan — Soudan — Sudán	—	—	—	—	—	—
Suriname	×	—	—	—	×	×
Sweden — Suède — Suecia	×	×	×	×	×	×
Switzerland — Suisse — Suiza	×	×	×	×	×	×

Table II. Receipt of statistics for 2023 *(continued)*
Tableau II. Réception des statistiques pour 2023 *(suite)*
Cuadro II. Recepción de las estadísticas de 2023 *(continuación)*

Country or territory Pays ou territoire País o territorio	Annual statistics Statistiques annuelles Estadísticas anuales	Quarterly statistics / Statistiques trimestrielles / Estadísticas trimestrales — Schedule II / Tableau II / Lista II				Reported consumption[a] La consommation déclarée[a] Consumo declarado[a]
		Q1	Q2	Q3	Q4	
Syrian Arab Republic — République arabe syrienne — República Árabe Siria	×	×	×	×	×	—
Tajikistan — Tadjikistan — Tayikistán	×	—	—	—	—	—
Thailand — Thaïlande — Tailandia	×	×	×	×	×	×
Timor-Leste[b]	×	×	—	×	×	×
Togo	×	—	—	—	—	—
Tonga	×	×	×	—	—	×
Trinidad and Tobago — Trinité-et-Tobago — Trinidad y Tabago	×	×	×	×	×	—
Tristan da Cunha — Tristán de Acuña	—	—	—	—	—	—
Tunisia — Tunisie — Túnez	×	×	×	×	×	—
Türkiye	×	×	×	×	×	×
Turkmenistan — Turkménistan — Turkmenistán	—	—	—	—	—	—
Turks and Caicos Islands — Îles Turques et Caïques — Islas Turcas y Caicos	×	×	×	×	×	×
Tuvalu[b]	—	—	—	—	—	—
Uganda — Ouganda	×	×	×	×	×	—
Ukraine — Ucrania	×	—	—	—	×	×
United Arab Emirates — Émirats arabes unis — Emiratos Árabes Unidos	×	×	×	×	×	×
United Kingdom — Royaume-Uni — Reino Unido	×	×	×	×	×	×
United Republic of Tanzania — République-Unie de Tanzanie — República Unida de Tanzanía	×	×	×	×	—	—
United States — États-Unis — Estados Unidos	×	×	×	×	×	×
Uruguay	×	×	×	×	×	×
Uzbekistan — Ouzbékistan — Uzbekistán	×	×	×	×	×	×
Vanuatu[b]	×	—	—	—	—	×
Venezuela (Bolivarian Rep. of) — Venezuela (Rép. bolivarienne du) — Venezuela (Rep. Bolivariana de)	×	×	×	—	×	×

Table II. Receipt of statistics for 2023 *(continued)*
Tableau II. Réception des statistiques pour 2023 *(suite)*
Cuadro II. Recepción de las estadísticas de 2023 *(continuación)*

Country or territory Pays ou territoire País o territorio	Annual statistics Statistiques annuelles Estadísticas anuales	Quarterly statistics / Statistiques trimestrielles / Estadísticas trimestrales — Schedule II / Tableau II / Lista II				Reported consumption[a] La consommation déclarée[a] Consumo declarado[a]
		Q1	Q2	Q3	Q4	
Viet Nam	—	—	—	—	—	—
Wallis and Futuna Islands — Îles Wallis-et-Futuna — Islas Wallis y Futuna	—	—	—	—	—	—
Yemen — Yémen	—	—	—	—	—	—
Zambia — Zambie	×	×	×	×	×	—
Zimbabwe	×	×	×	×	×	—

[a] Requested on a voluntary basis, pursuant to Commission on Narcotic Drugs resolution 54/6. — Ces renseignements sont demandés à titre volontaire, pour permettre à l'OICS d'appliquer la résolution 54/6 de la Commission des stupéfiants. — Esta información se solicita con carácter voluntario, de conformidad con la resolución 54/6 de la Comisión de Estupefacientes.

[b] Non-party to the 1971 Convention. — Non-partie à la Convention de 1971. — No parte en el Convenio de 1971.

[c] Statistics included in the report of Italy. — Statistiques incluses dans celles de l'Italie. — Las estadísticas han sido incluidas en el informe de Italia.

[d] Statistics included in the report of Switzerland. — Statistiques incluses dans celles de la Suisse. — Las estadísticas han sido incluidas en el informe de Suiza.

[e] Statistics included in the report of France. — Statistiques incluses dans celles de la France. — Las estadísticas han sido incluidas en el informe de Francia.

Table III. Defined daily doses for statistical purposes (S-DDD) for psychotropic substances in Schedules II, III and IV, by substance group and schedule

The term "defined daily doses for statistical purposes (S-DDD)", which has replaced the term "defined daily doses (DDD)", is used by INCB as a technical unit of measurement for the purpose of statistical analysis and is not a recommended prescription dose. Its definition is not free of a certain degree of arbitrariness. Certain psychotropic substances may be used in certain countries for different treatments or in accordance with different medical practices, and therefore a different daily dose could be more appropriate. The indicated S-DDD should be considered approximate and subject to modifications if more precise information becomes available. The basis for the grouping of the substances was, as far as possible, the anatomical therapeutic chemical classification system used in the Nordic Statistics on Medicines and recommended by the World Health Organization for drug utilization studies. In addition, the grouping reflects the Schedules of the 1971 Convention.

Tableau III. Doses quotidiennes déterminées à des fins statistiques (S-DDD) pour les substances psychotropes inscrites aux Tableaux II, III et IV, par groupe de substances et tableau

Le terme "doses quotidiennes déterminées à des fins statistiques (S-DDD)" remplace le terme "doses quotidiennes déterminées" utilisé par l'OICS. La S-DDD est une unité de mesure technique utilisée aux fins de l'analyse statistique et non une recommandation posologique. Sa définition n'est pas dépourvue d'un certain caractère arbitraire. Certaines substances psychotropes pouvant être utilisées pour différents traitements ou conformément à des pratiques médicales différentes dans différents pays, une autre dose quotidienne pourrait être mieux adaptée. Les S-DDD indiquées devraient être considérées comme approximatives et sujettes à modification si des indications plus précises venaient à être disponibles. Pour le regroupement des substances, on s'est fondé, dans la mesure du possible, sur le système de classification anatomique, thérapeutique et chimique utilisé dans les statistiques nordiques des médicaments et recommandé par l'Organisation mondiale de la santé pour les études sur l'utilisation des médicaments. En outre, ce regroupement correspond aux tableaux de la Convention de 1971.

Cuadro III. Dosis diarias definidas con fines estadísticos (S-DDD) para las sustancias sicotrópicas de las Listas II, III y IV, por grupo de sustancias y lista

La expresión "dosis diarias definidas" utilizada anteriormente por la JIFE fue sustituida por la expresión "dosis diarias definidas con fines estadísticos (S-DDD)". La S-DDD es una unidad técnica de medida que se utiliza a efectos del análisis estadístico, y no una dosis de prescripción recomendada. Su definición no está exenta de cierto grado de arbitrariedad. Es posible que determinadas sustancias se utilicen en determinados países para tratamientos diferentes o conforme a prácticas médicas diferentes y que, por lo tanto, resulte más apropiada otra dosis diaria. Las S-DDD que se indican deben considerarse aproximadas y podrían modificarse si se contara con información más precisa. En la medida de lo posible, las sustancias se agruparon con arreglo al sistema de clasificación anatómica, terapéutica y química utilizado en las estadísticas nórdicas sobre medicamentos y recomendado por la Organización Mundial de la Salud para los estudios sobre utilización de medicamentos. Además, es la forma en que están agrupadas en las listas del Convenio de 1971.

Table III. Defined daily doses for statistical purposes (S-DDD) for psychotropic substances in Schedules II, III and IV, by substance group and schedule

Tableau III. Doses quotidiennes déterminées à des fins statistiques (S-DDD) pour les substances psychotropes inscrites aux Tableaux II, III et IV, par groupe de substances et tableau

Cuadro III. Dosis diarias definidas con fines estadísticos (S-DDD) para las sustancias sicotrópicas de las Listas II, III y IV, por grupo de sustancias y lista

	S-DDD (mg)
Stimulants. Estimulantes	
A. Amphetamines in Schedule II / Amphétamines au Tableau II / Anfetaminas de la Lista II	
Amfetamine — Amfétamine — Anfetamina	15.00
Dexamfetamine — Dexamfétamine — Dexanfetamina	15.00
Levamfetamine — Lévamfétamine — Levanfetamina	15.00
Levomethamphetamine — Lévométhamphétamine — Levometanfetamina	15.00
Metamfetamine — Métamfétamine — Metanfetamina	15.00
Metamfetamine racemate — Racémate de métamfétamine — Racemato de metanfetamina	15.00
B. Other stimulants in Schedule II / Autres stimulants au Tableau II / Otros estimulantes de la Lista II	
4-Bromo-2,5-dimethoxyphenethylamine (2C-B) — 4-Bromo-2,5-diméthoxyphénéthylamine — 4-Bromo-2,5-dimetoxifenetilamina	—
Fenetylline — Fénétylline — Fenetilina	50.00
Methylphenidate — Méthylphénidate — Metilfenidato	30.00
Phencyclidine (PCP) — Fenciclidina (PCP)	—
Phenmetrazine — Phenmétrazine — Fenmetracina	50.00
C. Stimulants in Schedule III / Stimulants au Tableau III / Estimulantes de la Lista III	
Cathine — Catina	20.00
D. Stimulants in Schedule IV / Stimulants au Tableau IV / Estimulantes de la Lista IV	
Amfepramone — Amfépramone — Anfepramona	75.00
Aminorex	—
Benzfetamine — Benzfétamine — Benzfetamina	75.00
Etilamfetamine — Étilamfétamine — Etilanfetamina	30.00
Fencamfamin — Fencamfamine — Fencanfamina	80.00
Fenproporex	20.00
Mazindol	1.00
Mefenorex — Méfénorex	60.00
Mesocarb — Mésocarbe — Mesocarbo	25.00
Pemoline — Pémoline — Pemolina	40.00
Phendimetrazine — Phendimétrazine — Fendimetracina	70.00
Phentermine — Fentermina	15.00
Pipradrol	30.00
Pyrovalerone — Pyrovalérone — Pirovalerona	40.00

	S-DDD (mg)
Sedative-hypnotics. Sédatifs hypnotiques. Sedantes-hipnóticos	
E. Barbiturates in Schedule III and secobarbital (Schedule II) / Barbituriques au Tableau III et sécobarbital (Tableau II) / Barbitúricos de la Lista III y secobarbital (Lista II)	
Amobarbital	100.00
Butalbital	100.00
Cyclobarbital — Ciclobarbital	200.00
Pentobarbital	100.00
Secobarbital — Sécobarbital	100.00
F. Barbiturates in Schedule IV / Barbituriques au Tableau IV / Barbitúricos de la Lista IV	
Allobarbital — Alobarbital	100.00
Barbital	500.00
Butobarbital	150.00
Secbutabarbital	75.00
Vinylbital — Vinilbital	150.00
G. Benzodiazepines / Benzodiazépines / Benzodiazepinas	
Brotizolam	0.25
Estazolam	2.00
Flunitrazepam — Flunitrazépam	1.00
Flurazepam — Flurazépam	30.00
Haloxazolam	7.50
Loprazolam	1.00
Lormetazepam — Lormétazépam	1.00
Midazolam	15.00
Nimetazepam — Nimétazépam	5.00
Nitrazepam — Nitrazépam	5.00
Temazepam — Témazépam	20.00
Triazolam	0.25
H. Other sedative-hypnotics in Schedule III / Autres sédatifs-hypnotiques au Tableau III / Otros sedantes-hipnóticos de la Lista III	
Glutethimide — Glutéthimide — Glutetimida	250.00
I. Other sedative-hypnotics in Schedule IV / Autres sédatifs hypnotiques au Tableau IV / Otros sedantes hipnóticos de la Lista IV	
Ethchlorvynol — Etclorvinol	500.00
Ethinamate — Éthinamate — Etinamato	500.00
Methyprylon — Méthyprylone — Metiprilona	200.00
Zolpidem	10.00

Table III. Defined daily doses for statistical purposes (S-DDD) for psychotropic substances in Schedules II, III and IV, by substance group and schedule *(continued)*

Tableau III. Doses quotidiennes déterminées à des fins statistiques (S-DDD) pour les substances psychotropes inscrites aux Tableaux II, III et IV, par groupe de substances et tableau *(suite)*

Cuadro III. Dosis diarias definidas con fines estadísticos (S-DDD) para las sustancias sicotrópicas de las Listas II, III y IV, por grupo de sustancias y lista *(continuación)*

	S-DDD (mg)
J. Other sedative-hypnotics in Schedule II except secobarbital / Autres sédatifs-hypnotiques au Tableau II à l'exception du sécobarbital / Otros sedantes-hipnóticos de la Lista II con excepción del secobarbital	
Gamma-Hydroxybutyric acid (GHB) — Acide *gamma*-hydroxibutirique (GHB) — Ácido *gamma*-hidroxibutírico (GHB)	7500.00
Mecloqualone — Mécloqualone — Meclocualona	200.00
Methaqualone — Méthaqualone — Metacualona	200.00
Anxiolytics. Anxiolytiques. Ansiolíticos	
K. Benzodiazepines / Benzodiazépines / Benzodiazepinas	
Alprazolam	1.00
Bromazepam — Bromazépam	10.00
Camazepam — Camazépam	30.00
Chlordiazepoxide — Chlordiazépoxide — Clordiazepóxido	30.00
Clobazam	20.00
Clorazepate — Clorazépate — Clorazepato	20.00
Clotiazepam — Clotiazépam	15.00
Cloxazolam	9.00
Delorazepam — Délorazépam	3.00
Diazepam — Diazépam	10.00
Etizolam[a] — Étizolam[a]	—
Ethyl loflazepate — Loflazépate d'éthyle — Loflazepato de etilo	2.00
Fludiazepam — Fludiazépam	0.75
Halazepam — Halazépam	100.00
Ketazolam — Kétazolam	30.00
Lorazepam — Lorazépam	2.50
Medazepam — Médazépam	20.00
Nordazepam — Nordazépam	15.00
Oxazepam — Oxazépam	50.00
Oxazolam	40.00
Pinazepam — Pinazépam	15.00
Phenazepam — Phénazépam — Fenazepam	—
Prazepam — Prazépam	30.00
Tetrazepam — Tétrazépam	100.00
L. Other anxiolytics / Autres anxiolytiques / Otros ansiolíticos	
Meprobamate — Méprobamate — Meprobamato	1 200.00
Anti-epileptics. Antiépileptiques. Antiepilépticos	
M. Barbiturates / Barbituriques / Barbitúricos	
Methylphenobarbital — Méthylphénobarbital — Metilfenobarbital	100.00
Phenobarbital — Phénobarbital — Fenobarbital	100.00
N. Benzodiazepines / Benzodiazépines / Benzodiazepinas	
Clonazepam — Clonazépam	4.00
Analgesics. Analgésiques. Analgésicos	
O. Analgesics / Analgésiques / Analgésicos	
Buprenorphine — Buprénorphine — Buprenorfina	8.00
Lefetamine (SPA) — Léfétamine (SPA) — Lefetamina (SPA)	75.00
Pentazocine — Pentazocina	200.00
Anti-emetics. Antiémétiques. Antieméticos	
P. Anti-emetics / Antiémétiques / Antieméticos	
Delta-9-Tetrahydrocannabinol (*delta-9*-THC) and its stereochemical variants — *Delta-9*-Tétrahydrocannabinol et ses variantes stéréochimiques — *Delta-9*-Tetrahidrocannabinol y sus variantes estereoquímicas	30.00
Antitussives. Antitussifs. Antitusígenos	
Q. Antitussives / Antitussifs / Antitusígenos	
Zipeprol — Zipéprol	200.00
Antidepressants. Antidépresseurs. Antidepresivos	
R. Antidepressants / Antidépresseurs / Antidepresivos	
Amineptine — Amineptina	—

Table III. Defined daily doses for statistical purposes (S-DDD) for psychotropic substances in Schedules II, III and IV, by substance group and schedule *(continued)*

Tableau III. Doses quotidiennes déterminées à des fins statistiques (S-DDD) pour les substances psychotropes inscrites aux Tableaux II, III et IV, par groupe de substances et tableau *(suite)*

Cuadro III. Dosis diarias definidas con fines estadísticos (S-DDD) para las sustancias sicotrópicas de las Listas II, III y IV, por grupo de sustancias y lista *(continuación)*

New Psychoactive Substances (NPS) controlled under the 1971 Convention. Nouvelles substances psychoactive (NSP) placées sous contrôle au titre de la Convention de 1971. Nuevas sustancias psicoactivas (NSP) sometidas a fiscalización en virtud del Convenio de 1971.

S. NPS in Schedule II
NSP du Tableau II
NSP en la Lista II

	S-DDD (mg)
3,4-methylenedioxypyrovalerone (MDPV) — 3,4-méthylènedioxypyrovalérone (MDPV) — 3,4-metilendioxipirovalerona (MDPV)	—
3-methoxyphencyclidine — 3-méthoxyphencyclidine — 3-metoxifenciclidina	—
3-methylmethcathinone[a] — 3-méthylméthcathinone[a] — 3-metilmetcatinona[a]	—
4-Methylethcathinone (4-MEC) — 4-Méthylethcathinone (4-MEC) — 4-Metiletcatinona (4-MEC)	—
4-CMC (4-chloromethcathinone; clephedrone) — 4-CMC (4-chlorométhcathinone, cléphédrone) — 4-CMC (4-clorometcatinona, clefedrona)	—
4-F-MDMB-BINACA	—
5F-AMB-PINACA (5F-AMB, 5F-MMB-PINACA)	—
5F-MDMB-PICA (5F-MDMB-2201)	—
Alpha-Pyrrolidinovalerophenone (α-PVP) — *Alpha*-Pyrrolidinovalérophénone (α-PVP) — *Alfa*-Pirrolidinovalerofenona (α-PVP)	—
Alpha-PHP — *Alfa*-PHP	—
Alpha-PiHP[a]	—
AB-FUBINACA	—
ADB-BUTINACA[a]	—
AM-2201	—
5F-APINACA	—
CUMYL-PEGACLONE — CUMIL-PEGACLONE	—
Diphenidine — Diphénidine — Difenidina	—
Ethylone — Éthylone — Etilona	—
Ethylphenidate — Éthylphénidate — Etilfenidato	—
Eutylone[a] — Eutilona[a]	—
JWH-018	—
MDMB-4en-PINACA	—
MDMB-CHMICA	—
Mephedrone (4-methylmethcathinone) — Méphédrone (4-méthylméthcathinone) — Mefedrona (4-metilmetcatinona)	—
Methiopropamine (MPA) — Méthiopropamine (MPA) — Metiopropamina (MPA)	—
Methoxetamine (MXE) — Méthoxétamine (MXE) — Metoxetamina (MXE)	—
Methylone (*beta*-keto-MDMA) — Méthylone (bk-MDMA) — Metilona (*beta*-ceto-MDMA)	—
N-Benzylpiperazine (BZP) — *N*-Benzylpipérazine (BZP) — *N*-Bencilpiperazina (BZP)	—
Para-Methyl-4-methylaminorex (4,4'-DMAR) — Para-Méthyl-4-méthylaminorex (4,4'-DMAR) — Para-Metil-4-metilaminorex (4,4'-DMAR)	—
N-Ethylhexedrone — *N*-Éthylhexédrone — *N*-Etilhexedrona	—
Pentedrone — Pentédrone — Pentedrona	—
XLR-11	—

T. NPS in Schedule IV
NSP du Tableau IV
NSP en la Lista IV

	S-DDD (mg)
Clonazolam	—
Diclazepam — Diclazépam	—
Flualprazolam	—
Flubromazolam	—

Note: A dash (—) indicates that the substance has no assigned S-DDD. — *Note:* Un tiret (—) indique qu'il n'a pas été fixé de S-DDD pour la substance en question. — *Nota:* La raya (—) indica que la sustancia no tiene asignada una S-DDD.

[a] By its decisions 66/5, 66/6 and 66/7, the Commission on Narcotic Drugs decided to include ADB-BUTINACA, alpha-PiHP and 3-methylmethcathinone in Schedule II of the 1971 Convention on Psychotropic Substances. In accordance with article 2, paragraph 7 of that Convention, the decisions became fully effective with respect to each Party on 13 November 2023. — Par ses décisions 66/5, 66/6 and 66/7, la Commission a décidé d'inscrire ADB-BUTINACA, alpha-PiHP et 3-méthylméthcathinone au tableau II de la Convention sur les substances psychotropes de 1971. Conformément au paragraphe 7 de l'article 2 de la Convention, ces décisions ont pris pleinement effet pour chaque Partie le 13 Novembre 2023. — En sus decisiones 66/5, 66/6 and 66/7, la Comisiónde Estupefacientes decidió incluir la ADB-BUTINACA, alpha-PiHP y 3-metilmetcatinona en la Lista II en la Lista IV del Convenio sobre Sustancias Sicotrópicas de 1971. De conformidad con el artículo 2, párrafo 7, del Convenio, dichas decisiones surtieron pleno efecto respecto de cada una de las partes el 13 de Noviembre de 2023.

Table IV. Prohibition of and restrictions on export and import pursuant to article 13 of the Convention on Psychotropic Substances of 1971

The Secretary-General has transmitted to all Governments notifications concerning the prohibition of the importation of specific substances in Schedules II, III and IV of the Convention on Psychotropic Substances of 1971 that were received from the countries indicated in the table below. The notifications are presented as follows: notifying countries listed alphabetically, followed by the prohibited substances and dates of notification.

The prohibitions are effective, with respect to exporting countries, as of the date of receipt of the Secretary-General's notification. Upon notification of a prohibition, an exporting country must take measures to ensure that none of the substances specified in the notification are exported to the country or any of the regions in the notifying country. Exports of a prohibited substance may be permitted only when a special import licence has been issued by the notifying country, in accordance with the provisions of article 13 of the 1971 Convention.

Tableau IV. Interdiction et restrictions à l'exportation et à l'importation conformément à l'article 13 de la Convention sur les substances psychotropes de 1971

Le Secrétaire général a transmis à tous les gouvernements des notifications reçues des pays énumérés dans le tableau ci-après concernant l'interdiction d'importer certaines substances figurant aux Tableaux II, III et IV de la Convention sur les substances psychotropes de 1971. Les notifications sont présentées de la façon suivante: pays ayant fait une notification, classés par ordre alphabétique, suivis des substances interdites et de la date de la notification. Les interdictions prennent effet pour les pays exportateurs à la date de réception de la communication émanant du Secrétaire général.

Au reçu d'une notification d'interdiction, les autorités des pays exportateurs doivent prendre les mesures nécessaires pour s'assurer qu'aucune des substances spécifiées dans ladite notification ne sera exportée vers le pays ayant fait la notification, ou vers une de ses régions. L'exportation d'une substance interdite ne peut être autorisée que si un permis spécial d'importation a été émis par l'autorité compétente du pays ayant fait la notification, conformément aux dispositions de l'article 13 de la Convention de 1971.

Cuadro IV. Prohibición y restricciones a la exportación e importación de conformidad con el artículo 13 del Convenio sobre Sustancias Sicotrópicas de 1971

El Secretario General ha transmitido a todos los gobiernos notificaciones recibidas de los países, que se indican en el cuadro siguiente, relativas a la prohibición de la importación de determinadas sustancias sicotrópicas de las Listas II, III y IV del Convenio sobre Sustancias Sicotrópicas de 1971. Las notificaciones se indican a continuación de la siguiente forma: países notificantes por orden alfabético seguidos de las sustancias prohibidas y las fechas de notificación. Las prohibiciones surtirán efecto, con respecto a los países exportadores, a partir de la fecha en que éstos reciban la notificación del Secretario General.

Al recibir una notificación de prohibición de importación, las autoridades de los países exportadores deberán tomar las medidas necesarias para asegurar que ninguna de las sustancias especificadas en la mencionada notificación sea exportada al país que ha hecho la notificación ni a ninguna de sus regiones. La exportación de una sustancia prohibida puede ser autorizada solamente si las autoridades competentes del país que ha hecho la notificación emiten un permiso especial de importación con arreglo a las disposiciones del artículo 13 del Convenio de 1971.

Table IV. Prohibition of and restrictions on export and import pursuant to article 13 of the Convention on Psychotropic Substances of 1971

Tableau IV. Interdiction et restrictions à l'exportation et à l'importation conformément à l'article 13 de la Convention sur les substances psychotropes de 1971

Cuadro IV. Prohibición y restricciones a la exportación e importación de conformidad con el artículo 13 del Convenio sobre sustancias sicotrópicas de 1971

Country and prohibited substances Pays et substances interdites País y sustancias prohibidas	Date of notification Date de la communication Fecha de notificación
Argentina — Argentine	
Mecloqualone — Mécloqualone — Meclocualona	15/01/1987
Methaqualone — Méthaqualone — Metacualona	24/03/1982
Australia — Australie	
Methaqualone — Méthaqualone — Metacualona	08/08/1980
Belize — Belice	
Amfetamine — Amfétamine — Anfetamina	09/05/1989
Dexamfetamine — Dexamfétamine — Dexanfetamina	
Fenetylline — Fénétylline — Fenetilina	
Levamfetamine — Lévamfétamine — Levanfetamina	
Levomethamphetamine — Lévométhamphétamine — Levometanfetamina	
Mecloqualone — Mécloqualone — Meclocualona	
Metamfetamine — Métamfétamine — Metanfetamina	
Metamfetamine racemate — Racémate de métamfétamine — Racemato de metanfetamina	
Methaqualone — Méthaqualone — Metacualona	
Methylphenidate — Méthylphénidate — Metilfenidato	
Phencyclidine (PCP) — Fenciclidina (PCP)	
Phenmetrazine — Phenmétrazine — Fenmetracina	
Secobarbital — Sécobarbital	
Bulgaria — Bulgarie	
Amfetamine — Amfétamine — Anfetamina	12/08/1993
Dexamfetamine — Dexamfétamine — Dexanfetamina	
Fenetylline — Fénétylline — Fenetilina	
Levamfetamine — Lévamfétamine — Levanfetamina	
Metamfetamine — Métamfétamine — Metanfetamina	
Metamfetamine racemate — Racémate de métamfétamine — Racemato de metanfetamina	
Chile — Chili	
Glutethimide — Glutéthimide — Glutetimida	01/07/1981
Lefetamine (SPA) — Léfétamine (SPA) — Lefetamina (SPA)	
Mecloqualone — Mécloqualone — Meclocualona	
Methaqualone — Méthaqualone — Metacualona	
Phencyclidine (PCP) — Fenciclidina (PCP)	
Phenmetrazine — Phenmétrazine — Fenmetracina	
Colombia — Colombie	
Methaqualone — Méthaqualone — Metacualona	11/11/1981
Gabon — Gabón	
Methaqualone — Méthaqualone — Metacualona	28/07/1993
Iceland — Islande — Islandia	
Phencyclidine (PCP) — Fenciclidina (PCP)	28/11/1979
India — Inde	
Amfepramone — Amfépramone — Anfepramona	30/05/1991
Aminorex	27/10/2005
Benzfetamine — Benzfétamine — Benzfetamina	30/05/1991
Bromazepam — Bromazépam	
Brotizolam	27/10/2005
Camazepam — Camazépam	30/05/1991
Clorazepate — Clorazépate — Clorazepato	
Clotiazepam — Clotiazépam	
Cloxazolam	
Delorazepam — Délorazépam	
Estazolam	
Ethinamate — Éthinamate — Etinamato	
Ethyl loflazepate — Loflazépate d'éthyle — Loflazepato de etilo	
Fludiazepam — Fludiazépam	
Flunitrazepam — Flunitrazépam	
Haloxazolam	
Ketazolam — Kétazolam	
Lefetamine (SPA) — Léfétamine (SPA) — Lefetamina (SPA)	
Loprazolam	
Lormetazepam — Lormétazépam	
Medazepam — Médazépam	
Mesocarb — Mésocarbe — Mesocarbo	27/10/2005
Methaqualone — Méthaqualone — Metacualona	30/04/1993
Methyprylon — Méthyprylone — Metiprilona	30/05/1991
Nimetazepam — Nimétazepam	
Oxazolam	
Phendimetrazine — Phendimétrazine — Fendimetracina	
Phentermine — Fentermina	
Pinazepam — Pinazépam	
Pipradrol	
Prazepam — Prazépam	
Temazepam — Témazépam	
Tetrazepam — Tétrazépam	
Japan — Japon — Japón	
Amfetamine — Amfétamine — Anfetamina	31/01/1991
Dexamfetamine — Dexamfétamine — Dexanfetamina	
Levamfetamine — Lévamfétamine — Levanfetamina	
Levomethamphetamine — Lévométhamphétamine — Levometanfetamina	
Metamfetamine — Métamfétamine — Metanfetamina	
Metamfetamine racemate — Racémate de métamfétamine — Racemato de metanfetamina	

Table IV. Prohibition of and restrictions on export and import pursuant to article 13 of the Convention on Psychotropic Substances of 1971 *(continued)*

Tableau IV. Interdiction et restrictions à l'exportation et à l'importation conformément à l'article 13 de la Convention sur les substances psychotropes de 1971 *(suite)*

Cuadro IV. Prohibición y restricciones a la exportación e importación de conformidad con el artículo 13 del Convenio sobre sustancias sicotrópicas de 1971 *(continuación)*

Country and prohibited substances Pays et substances interdites País y sustancias prohibidas	Date of notification Date de la communication Fecha de notificación
Latvia — Lettonie — Letonia	
Amfetamine — Amfétamine — Anfetamina	07/11/1995
Cathine — Catina	
Dexamfetamine — Dexamfétamine — Dexanfetamina	
Etilamfetamine — Étilamfétamine — Etilanfetamina	
Fenetylline — Fénétylline — Fenetilina	
Fenproporex	
Levamfetamine — Lévamfétamine — Levanfetamina	
Mefenorex — Méfénorex	
Metamfetamine — Métamfétamine — Metanfetamina	
Metamfetamine racemate — Racémate de métamfétamine — Racemato de metanfetamina	
Phentermine — Fentermina	
Lebanon — Liban — Líbano	
Amfetamine — Amfétamine — Anfetamina	16/10/2000
Benzfetamine — Benzfétamine — Benzfetamina	21/08/2007
Cathine — Catina	16/10/2000
Delta-9-Tetrahydrocannabinol — *Delta*-9-Tétrahydrocannabinol — *Delta*-9-Tetrahidrocannabinol	
Dexamfetamine — Dexamfétamine — Dexanfetamina	
Fenetylline — Fénétylline — Fenetilina	
Flunitrazepam — Flunitrazépam	21/08/2007
Levamfetamine — Lévamfétamine — Levanfetamina	16/10/2000
Levomethamphetamine — Lévométhamphétamine — Levometanfetamina	
Mecloqualone — Mécloqualone — Meclocualona	
Metamfetamine — Métamfétamine — Metanfetamina	
Metamfetamine racemate — Racémate de métamfétamine — Racemato de metanfetamina	
Methaqualone — Méthaqualone — Metacualona	
Phencyclidine (PCP) — Fenciclidina (PCP)	
Triazolam	21/08/2007
Lithuania — Lituanie — Lituania	
Amfetamine — Amfétamine — Anfetamina	29/08/1997
Cathine — Catina	
Dexamfetamine — Dexamfétamine — Dexanfetamina	
Fenetylline — Fénétylline — Fenetilina	
Levamfetamine — Lévamfétamine — Levanfetamina	
Metamfetamine — Métamfétamine — Metanfetamina	
Metamfetamine racemate — Racémate de métamfétamine — Racemato de metanfetamina	
Madagascar	
Methaqualone — Méthaqualone — Metacualona	15/12/1978
Nigeria — Nigéria	
Amfetamine — Amfétamine — Anfetamina	27/02/1986
Dexamfetamine — Dexamfétamine — Dexanfetamina	
Metamfetamine — Métamfétamine — Metanfetamina	
Methaqualone — Méthaqualone — Metacualona	
Methylphenidate — Méthylphénidate — Metilfenidato	
Pemoline — Pémoline — Pemolina	29/10/1990
Phencyclidine (PCP) — Fenciclidina (PCP)	27/02/1986
Phenmetrazine — Phenmétrazine — Fenmetracina	
Secobarbital — Sécobarbital	
Pakistan — Pakistán	
Amfepramone — Amfépramone — Anfepramona	06/12/1985
Amfetamine — Amfétamine — Anfetamina	
Barbital	
Benzfetamine — Benzfétamine — Benzfetamina	
Camazepam — Camazépam	
Clotiazepam — Clotiazépam	
Cloxazolam	
Cyclobarbital — Ciclobarbital	
Delorazepam — Délorazépam	
Dexamfetamine — Dexamfétamine — Dexanfetamina	
Ethchlorvynol — Etclorvinol	
Ethinamate — Éthinamate — Etinamato	
Ethyl loflazepate — Loflazépate d'éthyle — Loflazepato de etilo	
Flunitrazepam — Flunitrazépam	
Flurazepam — Flurazépam	
Glutethimide — Glutéthimide — Glutetimida	
Halazepam — Halazépam	
Haloxazolam	
Lefetamine (SPA) — Léfétamine (SPA) — Lefetamina (SPA)	
Loprazolam	
Mazindol	
Mecloqualone — Mécloqualone — Meclocualona	
Metamfetamine — Métamfétamine — Metanfetamina	
Methaqualone — Méthaqualone — Metacualona	
Methylphenobarbital — Méthylphénobarbital — Metilfenobarbital	
Methyprylon — Méthyprylone — Metiprilona	
Nordazepam — Nordazépam	
Oxazolam	
Phencyclidine (PCP) — Fenciclidina (PCP)	
Phendimetrazine — Phendimétrazine — Fendimetracina	
Phenmetrazine — Phenmétrazine — Fenmetracina	
Pipradrol	
Secobarbital — Sécobarbital	
Tetrazepam — Tétrazépam	
Peru — Pérou — Perú	
Lefetamine (SPA) — Léfétamine (SPA) — Lefetamina (SPA)	07/04/2005
Phendimetrazine — Phendimétrazine — Fendimetracina	08/04/2005

Table IV. Prohibition of and restrictions on export and import pursuant to article 13 of the Convention on Psychotropic Substances of 1971 *(continued)*

Tableau IV. Interdiction et restrictions à l'exportation et à l'importation conformément à l'article 13 de la Convention sur les substances psychotropes de 1971 *(suite)*

Cuadro IV. Prohibición y restricciones a la exportación e importación de conformidad con el artículo 13 del Convenio sobre sustancias sicotrópicas de 1971 *(continuación)*

Country and prohibited substances Pays et substances interdites País y sustancias prohibidas	Date of notification Date de la communication Fecha de notificación
Russian Federation — Fédération de Russie — Federación de Rusia	
Cathine — Catina	09/11/2005
Saudi Arabia — Arabie saoudite — Arabia Saudita	
Fenetylline — Fénétylline — Fenetilina	31/12/1987
Methaqualone — Méthaqualone — Metacualona	
Senegal — Sénégal	
Amfetamine — Amfétamine — Anfetamina	16/05/1980
Dexamfetamine — Dexamfétamine — Dexanfetamina	
Mecloqualone — Mécloqualone — Meclocualona	31/01/1991
Metamfetamine — Métamfétamine — Metanfetamina	16/05/1980
Methaqualone — Méthaqualone — Metacualona	
Methylphenidate — Méthylphénidate — Metilfenidato	
Phencyclidine (PCP) — Fenciclidina (PCP)	
Phenmetrazine — Phenmétrazine — Fenmetracina	
South Africa — Afrique du Sud — Sudáfrica	
Methaqualone — Méthaqualone — Metacualona	15/12/1978
Thailand — Thaïlande — Tailandia	
Amfetamine — Amfétamine — Anfetamina	15/08/1991
Dexamfetamine — Dexamfétamine — Dexanfetamina	
Fenetylline — Fénétylline — Fenetilina	
Levamfetamine — Lévamfétamine — Levanfetamina	
Levomethamphetamine — Lévométhamphétamine — Levometanfetamina	
Metamfetamine — Métamfétamine — Metanfetamina	
Phenmetrazine — Phenmétrazine — Fenmetracina	
Togo	
Amfetamine — Amfétamine — Anfetamina	28/07/1993
Ethinamate — Éthinamate — Etinamato	
Lefetamine (SPA) — Léfétamine (SPA) — Lefetamina (SPA)	
Mecloqualone — Mécloqualone — Meclocualona	
Metamfetamine — Métamfétamine — Metanfetamina	
Methylphenidate — Méthylphénidate — Metilfenidato	
Methylphenobarbital — Méthylphénobarbital — Metilfenobarbital	
Methyprylon — Méthyprylone — Metiprilona	
Pemoline — Pémoline — Pemolina	
Phencyclidine (PCP) — Fenciclidina (PCP)	
Pipradrol	
Secobarbital — Sécobarbital	
Türkiye	
Amfepramone — Amfépramone — Anfepramona	30/06/1981
Amfetamine — Amfétamine — Anfetamina	
Dexamfetamine — Dexamfétamine — Dexanfetamina	
Fenetylline — Fénétylline — Fenetilina	27/09/1999
Flunitrazepam — Flunitrazépam	
Metamfetamine — Métamfétamine — Metanfetamina	30/06/1981
Metamfetamine racemate — Racémate de métamfétamine — Racemato de metanfetamina	27/09/1999
Methaqualone — Méthaqualone — Metacualona	20/08/1982
Pemoline — Pémoline — Pemolina	27/09/1999
Phendimetrazine — Phendimétrazine — Fendimetracina	30/06/1981
Phenmetrazine — Phenmétrazine — Fenmetracina	
Phentermine — Fentermina	
Pipradrol	
United States — États-Unis — Estados Unidos	
Flunitrazepam — Flunitrazépam	09/10/1996
Methaqualone — Méthaqualone — Metacualona	09/09/1985
Venezuela (Bolivarian Republic of) — Venezuela (la République bolivarienne du) — Venezuela (República Bolivariana de)	
Amfetamine — Amfétamine — Anfetamina	02/06/1992
Dexamfetamine — Dexamfétamine — Dexanfetamina	
Levamfetamine — Lévamfétamine — Levanfetamina	
Levomethamphetamine — Lévométhamphétamine — Levometanfetamina	
Metamfetamine — Métamfétamine — Metanfetamina	
Metamfetamine racemate — Racémate de métamfétamine — Racemato de metanfetamina	
Methaqualone — Méthaqualone — Metacualona	22/05/1986
Phenmetrazine — Phenmétrazine — Fenmetracina	02/06/1992
Yemen — Yémen	
Amfetamine — Amfétamine — Anfetamina	18/11/1980
Ethinamate — Éthinamate — Etinamato	
Lefetamine (SPA) — Léfétamine (SPA) — Lefetamina (SPA)	
Metamfetamine — Métamfétamine — Metanfetamina	
Methaqualone — Méthaqualone — Metacualona	
Methylphenidate — Méthylphénidate — Metilfenidato	
Methylphenobarbital — Méthylphénobarbital — Metilfenobarbital	
Methyprylon — Méthyprylone — Metiprilona	
Phencyclidine (PCP) — Fenciclidina (PCP)	
Phenmetrazine — Phenmétrazine — Fenmetracina	
Pipradrol	

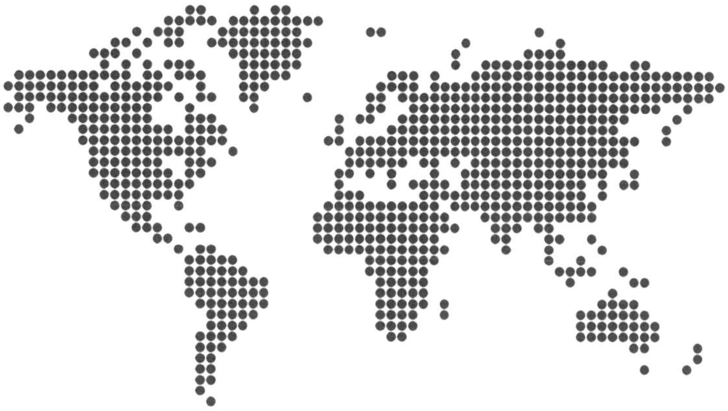

Part two
Deuxième partie
Segunda parte

COMMENTS ON THE REPORTED STATISTICS ON AND ASSESSMENTS OF PSYCHOTROPIC SUBSTANCES

Overview

The analysis contained in the present part of the technical publication on psychotropic substances is based on statistical data and assessment data furnished by Governments. The quality of the analysis depends on the quality of the data provided.

The first section of the analysis presents the main trends found in the data reported by countries and territories, beginning with an overview of the situation regarding the 170 psychotropic substances under international control in 2023, and highlights key trends identified in the data. It also provides updates on the status of the control of psychotropic substances and changes in scheduling under the Convention on Psychotropic Substances of 1971.

The first section continues with a comprehensive analysis of the substances that were of greatest interest in 2023. The analysis is broken down by drug family, beginning with tetrahydrocannabinol (THC) and *delta*-9-THC, the hallucinogens 3,4-methylenedioxymethamphetamine (MDMA), psilocybine and psilocine (psilotsin), followed by stimulants, benzodiazepines, barbiturates, other sedative-hypnotics, anxiolytics (specifically meprobamate) and buprenorphine. The most pertinent data related to manufacture, imports, exports, stocks and reported consumption are reviewed, and trends identified in the data for 2023 are compared with trends from previous years. Additional analyses and information are provided on substances used in the manufacture of exempted preparations.

The second section provides an analysis of the assessment system for psychotropic substances, including a review of global assessments reported by countries and territories.

All consumption data used have been provided by countries and territories as part of their annual statistical reports to the International Narcotics Control Board (INCB). Unless otherwise indicated, all consumption values are expressed in defined daily doses for statistical purposes (S-DDD) per 1,000 inhabitants per day, abbreviated $S\text{-}DDD_{ptpd}$. This unit of measure was adopted by the Board to measure the consumption of psychotropic substances in line with the approach taken by the World Health Organization Collaborating Centre for Drug Statistics Methodology.

The analysis contained in the present publication reflects only the most significant aspects of licit activity involving internationally controlled psychotropic substances. Complete data for 2023, including data on consumption, and assessments for 2025 can be found in electronic format on the INCB website.

English

TRENDS IN REPORTED DATA ON PSYCHOTROPIC SUBSTANCES

The situation with regard to psychotropic substances in 2023

1. As reflected in table II in the present publication, as at 1 November 2024, 163 countries and 14 territories had provided their annual statistical reports in accordance with article 16 of the Convention on Psychotropic Substances of 1971. Those figures represented an increase from the previous year, when 155 countries and 14 territories had provided their annual statistical reports by 1 November.

2. Reporting performance improved in all regions in 2023 compared with 2022. For 2023, at least 68 per cent of all countries and territories in each region provided the required annual statistical report (see table 1).

Table 1. Annual statistics reporting performance for countries and territories, by region, 2022 and 2023

	Number of countries and territories	
Region	*2022*	*2023*
Africa	39 out of 57 (68 per cent)	42 out of 57 (74 per cent)
Americas	36 out of 45 (80 per cent)	37 out of 45 (82 per cent)
Asia	40 out of 48 (83 per cent)	41 out of 48 (85 per cent)
Europe	41 out of 43 (95 per cent)	42 out of 43 (98 per cent)
Oceania	13 out of 22 (59 per cent)	15 out of 22 (68 per cent)

3. As at the end of 2023, 170 psychotropic substances had been placed under international control, up from 167 at the end of 2022. In March 2023, the Commission on Narcotic Drugs decided to include ADB-BUTINACA, *alpha*-PiHP and 3-methylmethcathinone in Schedule II of the 1971 Convention, and the substances came under international control in November 2023.

4. The psychotropic substances under international control comprise several drug categories and types and are used to treat an extensive number of health conditions. Most psychotropic substances manufactured and consumed are sedative-hypnotics, anxiolytics and anti-epileptics, including barbiturates and benzodiazepines. The other significant group manufactured comprises stimulants, mostly amphetamines and methylphenidate. The remaining substances that are regularly manufactured – hallucinogens, analgesics and anti-anaemics – account for only a small proportion of the overall manufacture of psychotropic substances.

5. Overall trends in the manufacture of psychotropic substances under international control remained largely consistent in 2023 as compared with 2022. In terms of gross weight, the substance most manufactured globally was phenobarbital, at 374 tons, a far larger quantity than for any other substance (see figure 1). Methylphenidate was the second most manufactured substance globally, at 82.6 tons, which, according to International Narcotics Control Board (INCB) data, was the largest amount of the substance ever manufactured worldwide in a single year. Manufacture of meprobamate had ranked second in 2022 but dropped significantly in 2023, as reported manufacture fell by more than half, to 39.5 tons.

6. When considered in terms of doses (S-DDD), the psychotropic substances manufactured in the largest quantities in 2023 present a different picture compared with the ranking by gross weight (see figure 2). In 2023, alprazolam was the most manufactured substance, at over 15.5 billion S-DDD, nearly triple the 5.8 billion S-DDD reported for diazepam, which was the second most manufactured substance. The other psychotropic substances manufactured in the highest quantities in 2023 in terms of doses were clonazepam (4.48 billion S-DDD), lorazepam (4.08 billion S-DDD), zolpidem (3.97 billion S-DDD), phenobarbital (3.74 billion S-DDD), dexamfetamine (3.18 billion S-DDD), methylphenidate (2.75 billion S-DDD), buprenorphine (1.94 billion S-DDD) and phentermine (1.77 billion S-DDD). In 2023, another 23 psychotropic substances were manufactured in quantities exceeding 100 million doses.

7. The primary countries manufacturing psychotropic substances generally remained the same as in previous years. In terms of gross weight, India was the largest manufacturer in 2023, as it is a primary manufacturer of

Figure 1. Most manufactured psychotropic substances worldwide, based on gross weight, 2023

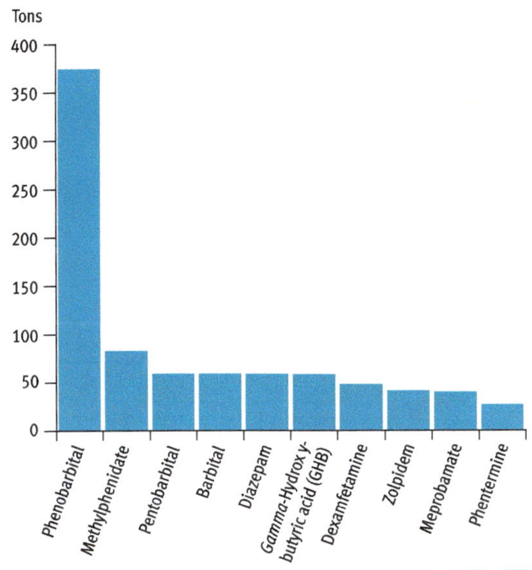

Figure 2. Most manufactured psychotropic substances worldwide, based on total S-DDD, 2023

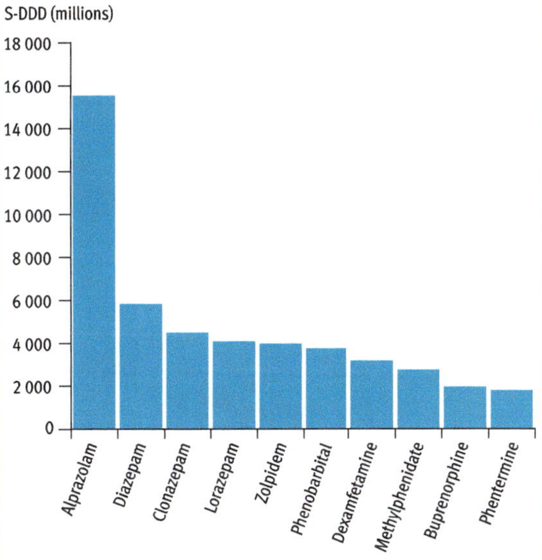

several barbiturates and benzodiazepines. China was the second largest manufacturer, mostly owing to its role as a major manufacturer of several barbiturates. The United States of America, Italy and Germany round out the top five manufacturers by gross weight. In terms of S-DDD, the top five countries were the same, but with Italy ranking second and China fourth. Notably, Switzerland, which historically reported much higher quantities of manufacture of psychotropic substances (more than 80 tons in 2018) has reported far less in the past few years (7.4 tons in 2023), mostly owing to the country ceasing manufacture of *gamma*-hydroxybutyric acid (GHB) and *N*-benzylpiperazine (BZP).

8. With regard to international trade, six benzodiazepines were among the most widely traded psychotropic substances in 2023 (see table 2). Phenobarbital was the most widely traded barbiturate under international control, while methylphenidate was the most widely traded stimulant. Zolpidem was the most traded non-benzodiazepine non-barbiturate sedative. The number of countries and territories reporting imports of buprenorphine continued to rise compared with previous years, although the volume of trade in the substance was lower in 2023 than in 2022.

Table 2. Most widely traded internationally controlled psychotropic substances, 2023

Substance	*S-DDD (mg)*	*Total imports (kg)*	*Total imports (millions of S-DDD)*	*Number of importing countries and territories*
Diazepam	10	37 180.25	3 718.02	164
Midazolam	15	8 551.21	570.08	159
Phenobarbital	100	208 219.59	2 082.20	158
Clonazepam	4	11 374.47	2 843.62	142
Alprazolam	1	14 904.43	14 904.43	139
Lorazepam	2.5	8 540.29	3 416.12	126
Methylphenidate	30	59 952.31	1 998.41	120
Zolpidem	10	35 814.82	3 581.48	118
Bromazepam	10	15 861.96	1 586.20	113
Buprenorphine	8	9 915.08	1 239.39	97

9. As in previous years, diazepam was the most widely imported internationally controlled psychotropic substance in 2023, with 164 countries and territories reporting imports of the substance totalling 37.2 tons, the lowest amount since 2017. Similarly, total imports for midazolam, phenobarbital and clonazepam in 2023 were 10 to

Figure 3. Most consumed psychotropic substances worldwide, based on total S-DDD, 2023

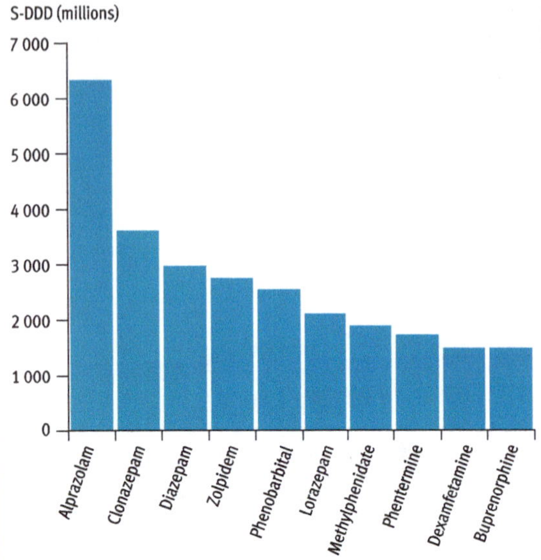

Figure 4. *Delta*-9-Tetrahydrocannabinol: manufacture and stocks, 2014–2023

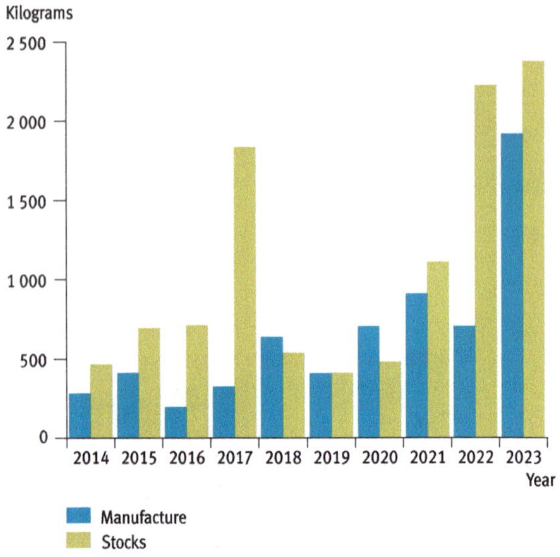

30 per cent lower than in 2022. Imports of alprazolam rose by nearly 50 per cent in 2023 compared with 2022. The other most widely traded substances did not see significant changes in the volumes imported in 2023 compared with 2022.

10. A total of 111 countries and territories (63 per cent of those that submitted their annual statistics) provided data regarding the consumption of at least one psychotropic substance in 2023, up from 100 countries and territories in 2022. Reporting rates at the regional level varied widely: data on consumption in 2023 were provided by 20 countries and territories in Africa (35 per cent of the total number of countries and territories in the region), 25 countries and territories in the Americas (56 per cent), 22 countries and territories in Asia (46 per cent), 35 countries and territories in Europe (81 per cent) and 9 countries and territories in Oceania (41 per cent).

11. As the S-DDD values established for psychotropic substances can vary greatly between different substances (see table III in the present publication), an analysis of consumption data by gross weight would not accurately reflect global consumption trends. Consumption data expressed in total S-DDD better reflect the consumption patterns in reporting countries and territories and lend themselves better to analysis. Figure 3 presents the most consumed psychotropic substances worldwide in 2023 in terms of total doses (S-DDD).

12. In 2023, alprazolam was the most consumed substance, at over 6.3 billion S-DDD worldwide, nearly 1.5 billion more than in 2022. Consumption of clonazepam more than doubled, from 1.6 billion S-DDD in 2022 to 3.6 billion S-DDD in 2023. Consumption of diazepam also increased, rising by approximately 1 billion S-DDD to nearly 3 billion S-DDD in 2023. The other most consumed substances in 2023 all saw consumption increases ranging from 5 to 50 per cent. In contrast, global consumption of estazolam declined sharply, dropping from more than 3.1 billion S-DDD in 2022 to 1.2 billion S-DDD in 2023.

Tetrahydrocannabinol and *delta*-9-tetrahydrocannabinol

13. Tetrahydrocannabinol (THC) is a cannabinoid that is found naturally in the cannabis plant but can also be chemically synthesized. All isomers of THC are included in Schedule I of the 1971 Convention except for the isomer *delta*-9-tetrahydrocannabinol (*delta*-9-THC), which is included in Schedule II. The licit use of THC and *delta*-9-THC has been limited since they were put under international control; however, licit activity involving these substances has been increasing in recent years, as more countries have authorized some preparations of *delta*-9-THC for medical use.

Table 3. Tetrahydrocannabinol and *delta*-9-tetrahydrocannabinol: total global licit manufacture and stocks, 2023

Substance	*Manufacture (kg)*	*Stocks (kg)*
Tetrahydrocannabinol (all isomers included in Schedule I)	66.24	31.00
Delta-9-Tetrahydrocannabinol	1 919.36	2 378.48

14. As shown in table 3, manufacture of THC remains very limited. As was the case in 2022, Australia (62.93 kg) accounted for most of the reported manufacture of the substance in 2023. Trade in THC is also very limited, with only a few countries reporting any imports or exports. Canada was the largest exporter in 2023, reporting 560.81 kg, while the United States was the largest importer, with 84.01 kg. The activity of those two countries accounted for nearly all trade in 2023, with only a few additional countries reporting small quantities imported or exported. Australia was the largest consumer of THC in 2023, with 46.99 kg in consumption reported. No other country that provided consumption data for THC reported more than a few grams consumed.[1]

BOX 1. TETRAHYDROCANNABINOL AND *DELTA*-9-TETRAHYDROCANNABINOL: REPORTING CHANGES IN 2024

Beginning in 2024, the International Narcotics Control Board advised Governments to revise their reporting procedures under the Single Convention on Narcotic Drugs of 1961 as amended by the 1972 Protocol and the Convention on Psychotropic Substances of 1971 for cannabis as well as cannabinoids derived using natural and synthetic processes.

The Board recommended that countries and territories no longer report the quantities of cannabis extracts or tinctures manufactured, traded, in stock, utilized or consumed under the 1961 Convention as amended. Rather, countries and territories should report any preparation or by-product obtained from cannabis in terms of the cannabinoids, namely tetrahydrocannabinol (THC) and *delta*-9-THC, that it contains, which are controlled under the 1971 Convention.

The Board has acknowledged that reporting of THC and *delta*-9-THC may be challenging for some countries and territories depending on their control or data-gathering systems. The quantity of THC isomers manufactured from natural materials can vary depending on the raw material and process used to extract those isomers.

15. With respect to *delta*-9-THC, licit activity involving the substance has grown significantly in the past several years as more and more countries have authorized the use of pharmaceutical products and other preparations containing the substance. The manufacture of *delta*-9-THC has varied in quantity since 2014 but has generally been on the rise since 2020, when a total of 706.4 kg was reported (see figure 4). In 2023, 1.92 tons of *delta*-9-THC were manufactured worldwide; the largest quantity was reported by the United Kingdom of Great Britain and Northern Ireland, at 602.8 kg, followed by South Africa (514.4 kg), Germany (443.4 kg), Australia (207.2 kg) and the United States (139.4 kg).

16. Manufacturers' stocks of *delta*-9-THC have also varied significantly between 2014 and 2023 but have grown significantly since 2020, when global manufacturers' stocks stood at 481.9 kg. Those stocks increased to 1.11 tons in 2021, then to 2.22 tons in 2022. For 2023, global manufacturers' stocks stood at 2.38 tons. The largest holder of stocks in 2023 was the United Kingdom, at 1.1 tons, followed by South Africa (426.5 kg), Germany (398.4 kg), the United States (313.1 kg) and Australia (98.3 kg). Another 14 countries reported stocks of *delta*-9-THC, but in very small quantities.

17. Consumption of *delta*-9-THC is reported by a limited number of countries; only seven countries provided data for 2023. Before 2022, consumption of *delta*-9-THC was relatively low, with no country reporting consumption

[1] The consumption of tetrahydrocannabinol (THC) can be expressed only in terms of gross weight, as no value has been established for the substance's defined daily dose for statistical purposes (S-DDD).

English

of more than 0.3 $S\text{-}DDD_{ptpd}$ consumed. Beginning in 2022, consumption increased, notably in Australia, which reported 0.62 $S\text{-}DDD_{ptpd}$ that year, while other reporting countries reported less than 0.3 $S\text{-}DDD_{ptpd}$. Consumption in 2023 rose sharply, as South Africa reported consumption for the first time (5.53 $S\text{-}DDD_{ptpd}$), the highest among all countries that reported consumption data, followed by Australia (2.05 $S\text{-}DDD_{ptpd}$), Portugal (0.17 $S\text{-}DDD_{ptpd}$), Austria (0.06 $S\text{-}DDD_{ptpd}$), Switzerland (0.05 $S\text{-}DDD_{ptpd}$) and the United Kingdom (0.05 $S\text{-}DDD_{ptpd}$).

Hallucinogens

MDMA

18. MDMA is a stimulant with empathogenic, entactogenic and mild hallucinogenic properties that is included in Schedule I of the 1971 Convention. Since MDMA was placed under international control in the mid-1980s, the licit use of the substance has mostly been for limited scientific and clinical research. In recent years, a few countries have authorized the use of MDMA in exceptional cases for specific trauma-related mental health conditions, including post-traumatic stress disorder.

19. Licit activity involving MDMA was limited from the time when the substance was placed under international control until 2019, when manufacture and consumption of the substance increased, probably as a result of increasing research into possible therapeutic applications. MDMA is manufactured in only a few countries, although the total manufacture of 25.54 kg reported for 2023 was the largest amount of the substance manufactured in the past 10 years. The United Kingdom reported manufacture of 22.34 kg of the substance, followed by Canada at 2.68 kg. Australia, Netherlands (Kingdom of the), Switzerland and the United States also reported very small quantities. Since increasing its manufacture of MDMA in 2020, the United Kingdom has also been the primary holder of stocks of the substance, with approximately 12 kg in stocks each year since 2021. Global stocks of MDMA stood at 17.01 kg in 2023 (see figure 5).

20. A total of 22 countries and territories reported imports of MDMA in 2023, but as in previous years, the quantities traded were very small. Exports of MDMA were also limited; Canada, the primary exporter, reported exports of 0.67 kg in 2023. Overall, trade in MDMA has remained largely unchanged over the past decade.

21. Total consumption of MDMA in 2023 amounted to 16.67 kg, nearly all of which was reported by the United Kingdom (15.87 kg).[2] Canada, Switzerland and Israel were the other primary consumers, at 0.24 kg, 0.21 kg and 0.18 kg, respectively.

Figure 5. MDMA: manufacture, stocks and consumption, 2014–2023

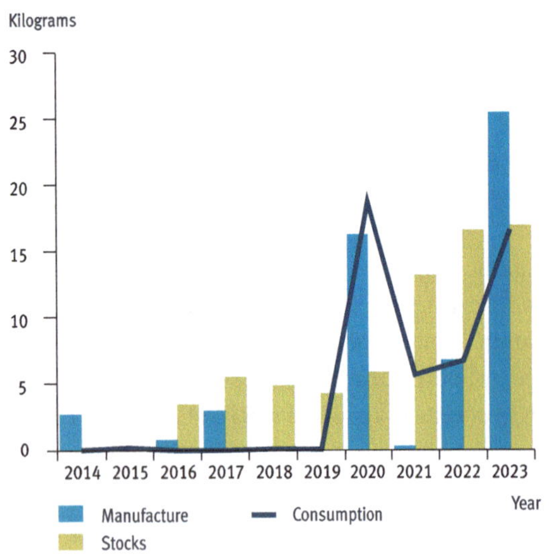

Figure 6. Manufacture of psilocybine and psilocine, 2014–2023

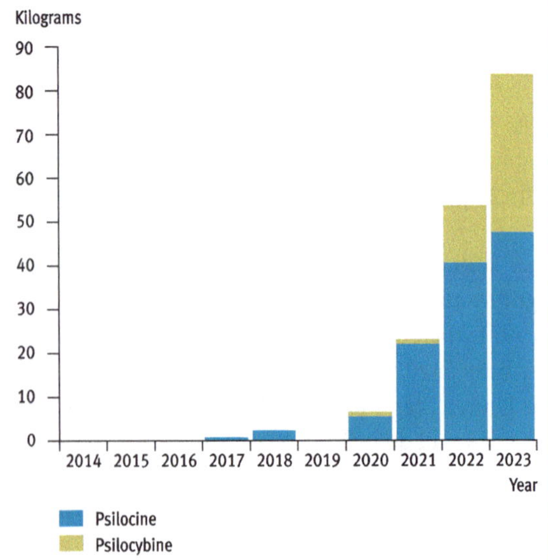

[2] The consumption of 3,4-methylenedioxymethamphetamine (MDMA) can be expressed only in terms of gross weight, as no S-DDD value has been established for the substance.

Psilocybine and psilocine

22. Psilocybine and psilocine (psilotsin) are hallucinogenic substances included in Schedule I of the 1971 Convention. Both substances occur naturally and can be found in many species of fungi in all parts of the world. Psilocybine is a prodrug that is converted into psilocine in the human body. As in the case of MDMA, licit activity involving psilocybine and psilocine has been very limited since they were placed under international control, but as more countries have authorized research and clinical trials involving the drugs, the licit manufacture of, trade in and consumption of those substances have increased in recent years.

23. Prior to 2020, the manufacture of psilocybine and psilocine was very limited, with total global manufacture not exceeding more than a few dozen grams. In 2020, total global manufacture of psilocybine increased to approximately 1 kg and changed only slightly in 2021. In 2022, total global manufacture increased to 13 kg, after which it increased further to 36.1 kg in 2023 (see figure 6). In 2022 and 2023, the United Kingdom was the primary manufacturer of psilocybine, reporting 8.9 kg and 30.9 kg, respectively. Canada, Netherlands (Kingdom of the) and the United States were the only other countries to report any significant manufacture in 2022 and 2023.

24. Like manufacture, trade in psilocybine and psilocine was very limited until 2020. Prior to 2020, the trade quantities reported by countries and territories rarely exceeded a few grams. In 2020, total global imports of psilocybine and psilocine stood at 0.46 kg and 0.04 kg, respectively. With regard to psilocybine, the figure rose to approximately 1 kg in 2021 and increased sharply in 2022, to 7.91 kg. In 2023, global imports of psilocybine remained steady at 7.8 kg. As for psilocine, total global imports rose to 0.04 kg in 2020 and have remained largely unchanged since then. In 2023, total global imports of the substance came to 0.06 kg.

25. Consumption of psilocine has not been reported by any country or territory in the past decade. Historically, consumption of psilocybine has been limited to no more than a few dozen grams reported by only a few countries. In 2022, global consumption rose significantly, to 1.3 kg, mainly as a result of increased consumption in the United Kingdom (0.64 kg), Germany (0.25 kg) and the United Sates (0.25 kg).[3] Total worldwide consumption of psilocybine further increased to 3.86 kg in 2023, with the United Kingdom (3.1 kg) accounting for the largest share, followed by the United States (0.46 kg) and Australia (0.13 kg). Another six countries reported consumption of the substance, but in only very small quantities.

Amphetamines

26. Six amphetamines are listed in Schedule II of the 1971 Convention: both optical isomers of amfetamine (levamfetamine and dexamfetamine) and their racemic mixture (amfetamine), and both optical isomers of metamfetamine (levomethamphetamine and metamfetamine) and their racemic mixture (metamfetamine racemate). Some of these substances, in particular dexamfetamine, are typically used to treat persons diagnosed with attention deficit hyperactivity disorder (ADHD).

27. Three amphetamines – amfetamine, dexamfetamine and metamfetamine – had a significant presence on the licit market in 2023, and 42 countries and territories imported at least one of them (see table 4). Of the three substances, the most manufactured was dexamfetamine. The global manufacture of dexamfetamine increased in 2023, mainly because of an increase in manufacture reported by the United States. Global manufacture of amfetamine was largely unchanged from 2022 to 2023, with the United States as the only manufacturer. With respect to metamfetamine, the quantity manufactured returned to 2021 levels after very little manufacture had been reported in 2022. Trade in the three substances increased between 2022 and 2023, driven mostly by increased imports of amfetamine and dexamfetamine reported by Germany.

[3] The consumption of psilocybine can be expressed only in terms of gross weight, as no S-DDD value has been established for the substance.

English

Table 4. Amphetamines with significant presence on the licit market: total global manufacture, imports and number of importing countries and territories, ranked by quantity manufactured, 2023

Substance	*S-DDD (mg)*	*Manufacture (kg)*	*Imports (kg)*	*Number of importing countries and territories*
Dexamfetamine	15	47 461.41	5 869.54	42
Amfetamine	15	16 766.23	835.63	31
Metamfetamine	15	596.89	1 200.37	24

Dexamfetamine

28. The total manufacture of dexamfetamine increased from 40 tons in 2022 to 47.5 tons in 2023 (see figure 7), as the United States reported an increase in manufacture of 10 tons compared with the previous year. As has been the case for many years, the United States was the largest manufacturer of dexamfetamine in 2023, at 42.6 tons. Other major manufacturers of the substance were Denmark (4.8 tons) and Finland (84.1 kg). France, which has historically been a major manufacturer of both dexamfetamine and amfetamine, has withdrawn from the market and not reported manufacture of any type of amphetamine since 2019.

29. Global imports of dexamfetamine have increased steadily over the past decade, rising from 1.79 tons in 2014 to 5.69 tons in 2023, with 41 countries and territories reporting imports in 2023. The largest importer was Germany, which reported 3.46 tons, followed by Australia (601.1 kg), Canada (505.9 kg), the Kingdom of the Netherlands (265.1 kg) and Chile (237 kg). The major importers of the substance thus remained unchanged compared with 2022. Total exports rose from 3.66 tons in 2022 to 4.41 tons in 2023, mostly owing to an increase in exports reported by Denmark, which led exports in 2023, at 3.08 tons, followed by France (449.8 kg), the United States (350.9 kg), Germany (326.1 kg) and Croatia (108.4 kg).

30. In 2023, 27 countries reported consumption of dexamfetamine. Overall consumption rose in most of those countries compared with the year before. Australia provided data on the consumption of the substance for the first time in 2023. Major consumers of dexamfetamine in 2023 were the United States (11.50 S-DDD_{ptpd}), Australia (4.25 S-DDD_{ptpd}), Israel (2.57 S-DDD_{ptpd}) and Canada (2.04 S-DDD_{ptpd}). All of the other countries that submitted consumption data reported rates below 2 S-DDD_{ptpd}. The 10 countries with the highest reported rates of consumption of dexamfetamine in 2023 are listed in table 5.

Figure 7. Dexamfetamine: global manufacture, imports and stocks, 2014–2023

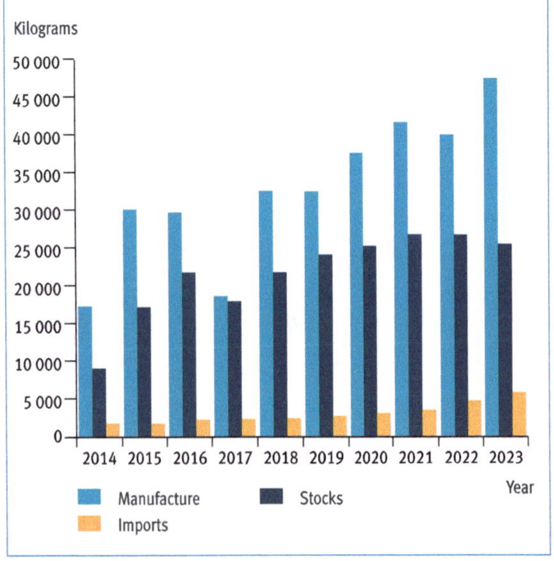

Figure 8. Dexamfetamine: quantities used in the manufacture of non-psychotropic substances, 2014–2023

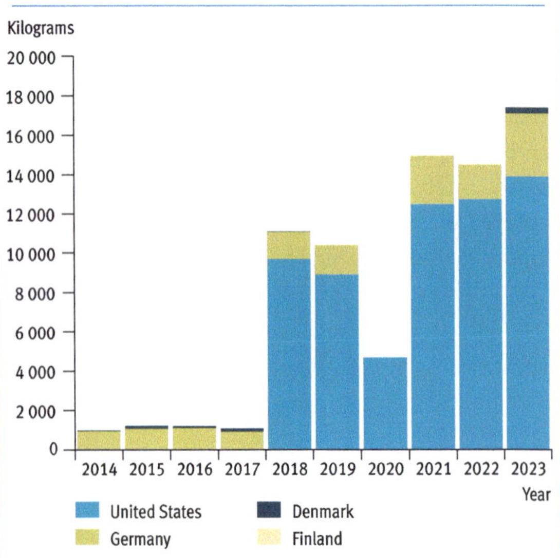

Table 5. Dexamfetamine: rates of consumption in the 10 countries reporting the highest consumption in 2023, compared with 2021 and 2022

	S-DDD per 1,000 inhabitants per day		
Country	*2021*	*2022*	*2023*
United States	8.57	8.05	11.50
Australia	–	–	4.25
Israel	1.52	2.07	2.57
Canada	1.60	1.90	2.04
Chile	0.53	0.78	1.58
Iceland	0.91	0.94	1.27
Netherlands (Kingdom of the)	1.10	1.26	1.26
Norway	–	1.00	1.14
Sweden	0.92	0.89	0.92
New Zealand	0.58	0.07	0.58

31. In the United States, dexamfetamine is also used in the synthesis of lisdexamfetamine (l-lysine-d-amfetamine), a prodrug of dexamfetamine that is not under international control and is used in the treatment of ADHD. The United States began reporting the use of dexamfetamine for the manufacture of non-psychotropic substances in 2018, and the quantity used has continued to grow since then. In 2023, 17.4 tons of dexamfetamine were used for the manufacture of non-psychotropic substances, mainly by the United States (13.9 tons). According to the information provided to the Board, that entire quantity was used for the manufacture of lisdexamfetamine. Germany and Denmark also reported the use of dexamfetamine for the manufacture of non-psychotropic substances in 2023, at 3.2 tons and 302 kg, respectively (see figure 8).

BOX 2. DEXAMFETAMINE PRODRUG: LISDEXAMFETAMINE

A prodrug is an inactive compound that becomes active once metabolized in the body, releasing its active drug component to exert its effects. One example is lisdexamfetamine (l-lysine-d-amfetamine), a prodrug of dexamfetamine, which is a central nervous system stimulant included in Schedule II of the Convention on Psychotropic Substances of 1971.

Lisdexamfetamine was pre-reviewed by the World Health Organization Expert Committee on Drug Dependence at its thirty-sixth meeting, in June 2014. In its report, the Committee stated that the safety and efficacy of lisdexamfetamine in the treatment of attention deficit hyperactivity disorder (ADHD) had been established. At the same time, the Committee concluded that the fact that lisdexamfetamine was a prodrug of dexamfetamine implied a need for similar clinical oversight and precautions for the monitoring and scheduling of this central nervous system stimulant. The substance never made it to the second step of the review process (critical review).

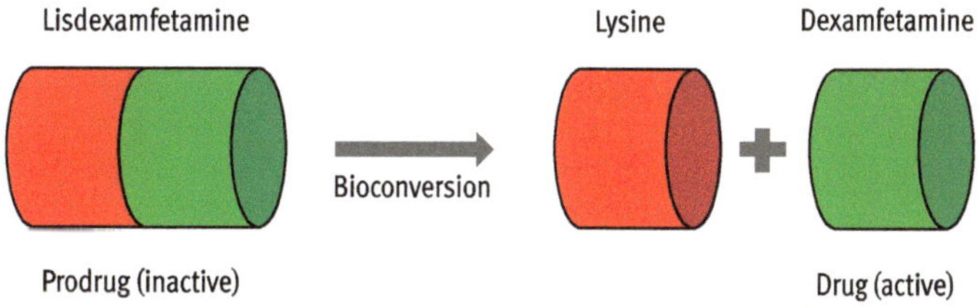

Primarily used in the treatment of ADHD, lisdexamfetamine has gained prominence since its commercialization in 2007 and has been marketed under various brand names, such as Vyvanse. When orally administered and metabolized in the human body, the substance is broken down into lysine, an amino acid, and dexamfetamine. Lisdexamfetamine has a lower potential for misuse compared with dexamfetamine and is not currently under international control; therefore, competent authorities are not obliged to monitor and report statistical data to the International Narcotics Control Board in the same manner as for psychotropic substances under international control. However, some countries do control the substance at the national level.

English

BOX 2. DEXAMFETAMINE PRODRUG: LISDEXAMFETAMINE *(continued)*

Recent data show an upward trend in the global manufacture of lisdexamfetamine, especially in the United States, which accounted for 90 per cent of global manufacture of dexamfetamine in 2023 and declared that 33 per cent of the substance had been used for the manufacture of lisdexamfetamine. Some European countries, including Denmark and Germany, have also seen an uptick in trade in dexamfetamine. Germany has reported increasing use of the substance for the manufacture of non-controlled psychotropic substances. The Board has also observed growing interest from Bolivia (Plurinational State of), Croatia and Panama regarding lisdexamfetamine.

As lisdexamfetamine is currently not under international control, the data available to the Board are provided by countries on a voluntary basis and therefore do not reflect the global situation. Nevertheless, on the basis of the data provided and enquiries received by various countries regarding lisdexamfetamine, it appears that the substance is gaining a significant presence on the licit international market. Over time, the consumption of dexamfetamine for medical purposes may be displaced by lisdexamfetamine.

The Board is grateful to the countries that have voluntarily shared information on lisdexamfetamine and encourages all countries and territories to share information on exports and imports of the substance in the future.

Amfetamine

32. The total manufacture of amfetamine increased by a small amount, from 16.1 tons in 2022 to 16.8 tons in 2023 (see figure 9). As in previous years, the United States was the main manufacturer of the substance, except for a few grams manufactured by several other countries. Global stocks of amfetamine fell from 22.5 tons in 2022 to 19.6 tons in 2023. Most of those stocks were held in the United States (19.2 tons). Canada was the other major holder of stocks and reported 257.9 kg. France, which historically held large stocks of amfetamine, reported a total of 12.4 kg for 2023.

33. Trade in amfetamine is relatively limited in comparison with the traded quantities of other psychotropic substances. Since 2018, imports of amfetamine have not exceeded 1 ton. For 2023, global imports of amfetamine stood at 835.6 kg, with Germany (560.7 kg) and Canada (239.3 kg) accounting for nearly all imports. Another 29 countries reported imports of the substance, but only in quantities of a few kilograms or less. As the primary manufacturer of amfetamine, the United States was the primary exporter of the substance, reporting 1.3 tons in 2023, up from 961.8 kg in 2022. Ten other countries also reported exports of amfetamine, but in quantities of only a few kilograms or less.

34. A total of 15 countries and territories reported consumption of amfetamine in 2023. Overall consumption increased slightly, mainly because of an increase in the United States, but many countries and territories reported lower consumption than in the previous year. The top five consuming countries and territories were the United States (10.51 S-DDD_{ptpd}), Canada (0.98 S-DDD_{ptpd}), the Turks and Caicos Islands (0.27 S-DDD_{ptpd}), Norway (0.10 S-DDD_{ptpd}) and Sweden (0.09 S-DDD_{ptpd}).

Metamfetamine

35. The global manufacture of metamfetamine increased from just a few grams reported in 2022 to 596.8 kg in 2023. Hungary reported manufacture of metamfetamine for the first time since 2020 and accounted for nearly all manufacture of the substance in 2023. Two other countries reported manufacture of a few grams of the substance. Global stocks of metamfetamine declined from 2.1 tons in 2022 to 243.5 kg in 2023, as France reported no stocks of the substance. Hungary accounted for nearly all global stocks.

36. For several years, trade in metamfetamine was minimal, with only a few grams imported or exported each year. In 2023, however, global imports and exports rose by 1.2 tons each, owing to the export of that quantity

Figure 9. Amfetamine: global manufacture, imports and stocks, 2014–2023

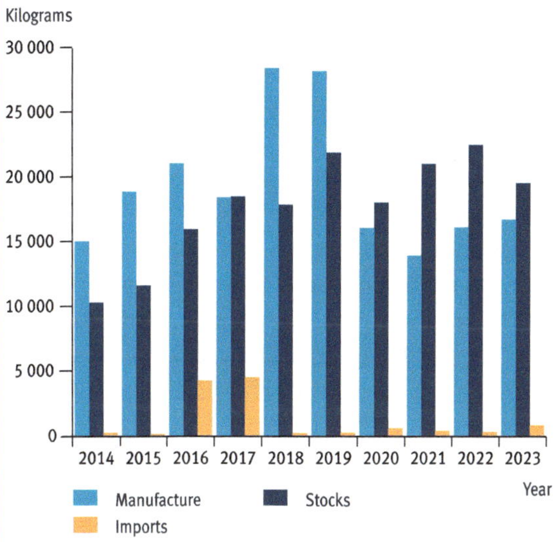

Figure 10. Methylphenidate: global manufacture, imports and stocks, 2014–2023

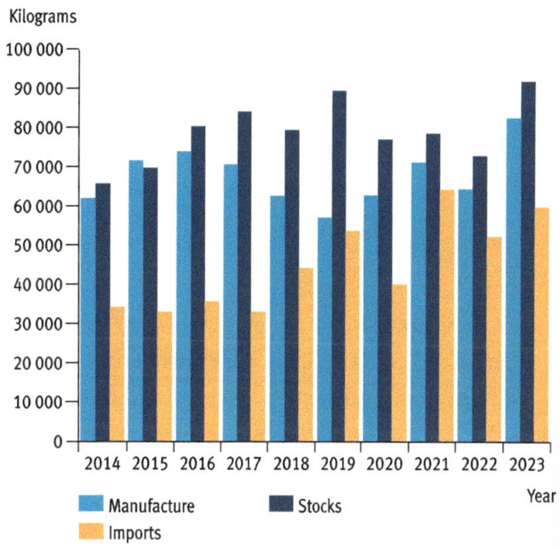

from France to the United States during that year. Other trade in metamfetamine remained limited, with a few other countries reporting exports and imports of just a few grams.

37. Consumption of metamfetamine is reported by only a few countries and in very low quantities. The only country to report any significant consumption in 2023 was North Macedonia (0.01 $\text{S-DDD}_{\text{ptpd}}$). New Zealand, which had reported some consumption in previous years, reported none in 2023.

Methylphenidate

38. Like amphetamines, methylphenidate is a stimulant included in Schedule II of the 1971 Convention and is also typically used for the treatment of ADHD. Among the stimulants included in Schedule II, it is the most widely manufactured and traded, with 120 countries and territories reporting imports of the substance in 2023 (see table 6).

Table 6. Methylphenidate: total global manufacture, imports and number of importing countries and territories, 2022 and 2023

Year	*S-DDD (mg)*	*Manufacture (kg)*	*Imports (kg)*	*Number of importing countries and territories*
2022	30	64 539.54	52 406.76	117
2023	30	82 645.73	59 952.31	120

39. The global manufacture of methylphenidate started to rise in 2012 and reached 74 tons in 2016, the highest level observed since the 1990s. Starting in 2017, worldwide manufacture of the substance exhibited a downward trend, dropping to 57.2 tons in 2019. Total manufacture then recovered and reached 82.6 tons in 2023, the highest level since INCB began receiving data (see figure 10).

40. Increases in the total manufacture of methylphenidate were mainly a result of increases reported by India, Switzerland and the United States. In 2023, the United States (58.4 tons) was again the leading manufacturer. India (11.2 tons), Switzerland (6.6 tons), the United Kingdom (4.7 tons) and Spain (1.1 tons) also manufactured significant quantities of the substance.

English

41. Global stocks of methylphenidate increased by nearly 20 tons, from 72.9 tons in 2022 to 92 tons in 2023. That increase can be attributed mostly to the United Kingdom, which increased its stocks from 2.9 tons to 17 tons, and to Germany, which increased its stocks from 6.8 tons to 8.9 tons. As in previous years, the United States (44.5 tons) accounted for nearly half of global stocks in 2023. The United Kingdom (17 tons), Germany (8.9 tons), Switzerland (7.6 tons) and Canada (4 tons) were the other major holders of stocks of methylphenidate.

42. International trade in methylphenidate remained highly active in 2023, with 120 countries and territories reporting imports of the substance and an increasing amount of the methylphenidate manufactured in the United States being exported to other countries.

43. The volume of imports of methylphenidate reported by countries and territories rose from 52.4 tons in 2022 to 60.0 tons in 2023. Most of the increase can be attributed to modest increases in imports by the leading importers. The five leading importers of methylphenidate in 2023 were Germany (10.5 tons), Canada (6.3 tons), Switzerland (5.8 tons), Spain (5.5 tons) and Belgium (3.5 tons). Another 13 countries imported more than 1 ton of the substance. Among the remaining countries and territories that reported imports of methylphenidate in 2023, 48 imported more than 10 kg of the substance.

44. The total volume of exports of methylphenidate reported by countries and territories increased from 49.8 tons in 2022 to 60.9 tons in 2023. The United States led in exports, at 17.4 tons, up from 15.8 tons in 2022. Other major exporters were Switzerland (9.1 tons), India (8.7 tons), the United Kingdom (6.1 tons), Germany (5.9 tons) and Spain (5.1 tons).

45. The use of methylphenidate for medical purposes increased significantly in the 1990s. The substance is used for the treatment of ADHD, primarily in children. It is also prescribed for the treatment of narcolepsy. The increase in the manufacture and use of methylphenidate was mainly the result of developments in the United States, where the substance is frequently prescribed for the treatment of ADHD and is also heavily advertised, including directly to potential consumers.

46. The number of countries and territories reporting methylphenidate consumption increased from 66 in 2022 to 80 in 2023. The difference between the highest and lowest rates of consumption remained considerable, mainly because of the significant quantity reported by Iceland, which has consistently exhibited high levels of consumption of methylphenidate for many years.

47. Compared with the figures reported for 2022, the consumption of methylphenidate in Iceland increased from 29.47 $S\text{-}DDD_{ptpd}$ to 34.50 $S\text{-}DDD_{ptpd}$; the country reported the highest consumption worldwide in 2023, as has been the case for many years. Consumption of the substance increased slightly in nearly all countries that provided data (see table 7).

Table 7. Methylphenidate: rates of consumption in the 10 countries reporting the highest consumption in 2023, compared with 2021 and 2022

	S-DDD per 1,000 inhabitants per day		
Country	*2021*	*2022*	*2023*
Iceland	53.33	29.47	34.50
Denmark	9.39	10.63	12.88
Canada	10.01	11.14	12.15
New Zealand	7.70	5.35	9.87
Sweden	8.57	9.01	9.61
Norway	—	8.38	9.14
Netherlands (Kingdom of the)	7.74	8.33	9.11
Israel	10.05	7.73	8.36
United States	7.34	6.90	7.14
Australia	—	—	6.38

Phentermine

48. Among the stimulants not included in Schedule II of the 1971 Convention, only one (phentermine) had any significant presence on the licit market in 2023. Phentermine has consistently remained the most manufactured non-amphetamine stimulant and is used medically as an appetite suppressant in the short-term management of obesity.

49. The volume of global manufacture of phentermine continued its decline in 2023, mainly because of reductions reported by Germany. The volume of imports of the substance rose in 2023 owing to a significant increase in imports by the United States. In total, 43 countries and territories reported imports of phentermine in 2023 (see table 8). Trends in consumption were largely unchanged, and New Zealand and Chile were the largest per capita consumers in 2023.

Table 8. Phentermine: total global manufacture and imports, 2023

Substance	*S-DDD (mg)*	*Manufacture (kg)*	*Imports (kg)*	*Number of importing countries and territories*
Phentermine	15	26 551.94	24 014.82	43

50. The global manufacture of phentermine dropped for a second year in a row, from 29.1 tons in 2022 to 26.6 tons in 2023, owing to a year-on-year reduction of 9 tons reported by the United States, while Germany reported an increase of 7 tons. Germany was the largest manufacturer of phentermine in 2023, at 19.3 tons, followed by the United States (3.7 tons), Italy (2.38 tons) and India (675.1 kg). Global stocks of phentermine also dropped for the second year in a row, from 27.5 tons in 2022 to 23.3 tons in 2023. The largest share of stocks was held by the United States (13.9 tons), followed by Germany (4.6 tons) and Italy (1 tons). Twenty-one other countries reported small stocks of the substance.

51. Global imports of phentermine rose in 2023, with 43 countries and territories reporting a total of 24 tons imported, up from 19.4 tons in 2022. As in 2022, the United States (9.2 tons) remained the leading importer of the substance, followed by Mexico (5 tons), Chile (2.7 tons) and the Republic of Korea (1.7 tons). Global exports of phentermine rose to 24.6 tons in 2023, with Germany remaining the top exporter of the substance (17 tons). Other major exporters included Italy (2.8 tons), Australia (962.4 kg), India (946.5 kg), Switzerland (888.6 kg) and the United States (887.5 kg).

52. Twenty-five countries and territories reported data on the consumption of phentermine in 2023, with New Zealand (14.35 $\text{S-DDD}_{\text{ptpd}}$), Chile (9.18 $\text{S-DDD}_{\text{ptpd}}$), the United States (8.56 $\text{S-DDD}_{\text{ptpd}}$), Mexico (8.31 $\text{S-DDD}_{\text{ptpd}}$) and the Republic of Korea (7.95 $\text{S-DDD}_{\text{ptpd}}$) reporting the highest rates of consumption, mirroring the top five from the year before. Although the countries with the highest consumption of phentermine remained unchanged from 2022, overall consumption decreased in all countries and territories in 2023.

Benzodiazepines

53. Benzodiazepines are a class of substances placed in Schedule IV of the 1971 Convention and used for the treatment of a range of conditions. Some of the most commonly prescribed benzodiazepines are used to treat anxiety, panic disorders, depression and insomnia, and some are also used for general anaesthesia, sedation prior to surgery, alcohol withdrawal and drug-associated agitation. Trade in benzodiazepines has been a global phenomenon for many decades. During the period 2014–2023, nearly all countries and territories reported trade in at least one benzodiazepine in a quantity of more than 1 kg to INCB.

54. In the early 1980s, benzodiazepines began to come under international control. Over time, control measures have been expanded to include additional substances, and currently 41 benzodiazepines are internationally controlled, including four that are classified as new psychoactive substances.

55. Of the 41 benzodiazepines under international control, 16 had a significant presence on the licit market in 2023 (see table 9). As in previous years, diazepam, midazolam, clonazepam, alprazolam and lorazepam were

English

the most widely traded benzodiazepines in 2023, with each substance imported by 126 or more countries and territories. In comparison with 2022, the number of countries and territories reporting imports of those benzodiazepines changed only slightly.

Table 9. Benzodiazepines with significant presence on the licit market: total global manufacture and number of importing countries and territories, ranked by manufacture in S-DDD, 2023

Substance	*S-DDD (mg)*	*Manufacture (kg)*	*Manufacture (millions of S-DDD)*	*Number of importing countries and territories*
Alprazolam	1	15 550.22	15 550.22	139
Diazepam	10	58 226.30	5 822.63	164
Clonazepam	4	17 938.95	4 484.74	142
Lorazepam	2.5	10 198.60	4 079.44	126
Bromazepam	10	8 959.04	895.90	113
Chlordiazepoxide	30	22 826.23	760.87	83
Midazolam	15	9 157.37	610.49	159
Nitrazepam	5	2 860.76	572.15	54
Flunitrazepam	1	543.73	543.73	31
Clobazam	20	8 734.77	436.74	95
Oxazepam	50	18 799.45	375.99	53
Temazepam	20	6 853.11	342.66	32
Triazolam	0.25	57.70	230.79	39
Prazepam	30	3 900.33	130.01	27
Flurazepam	30	2 757.74	91.92	21
Clorazepate	20	1 486.93	74.35	44

56. In 2023, the total reported manufacture of benzodiazepines with a significant presence on the licit market reached approximately 189 tons, marking an increase compared with 2022. While manufacture was reported in multiple regions around the world, 96 per cent of total manufacture was concentrated in four countries: Italy (41 per cent), India (37 per cent), China (9 per cent) and Brazil (9 per cent). Despite a slight decrease in manufacture, Italy remained the leading manufacturer. Manufacture in India increased by 31 per cent compared with 2022 and reached a record high, while China nearly doubled its manufacture from 2022 to 2023. In terms of gross weight, eight benzodiazepines – diazepam, chlordiazepoxide, oxazepam, clonazepam, alprazolam, lorazepam, midazolam and bromazepam – accounted for 86 per cent of total manufacture in 2023 (see figure 11).

Diazepam

57. Diazepam was the most manufactured benzodiazepine in 2023 in terms of gross weight (58.2 tons) and accounted for 31 per cent of the overall manufacture of benzodiazepines with a significant presence on the licit market. The global manufacture of diazepam has fluctuated markedly in recent years. Manufacture of the substance in Italy peaked at 29.2 tons in 2021 but then declined sharply, falling to 17.9 tons in 2023. In contrast, India increased its manufacture substantially, from 12.7 tons in 2022 to 20.9 tons in 2023. Manufacture in China has been volatile, dropping as low as 1.3 tons in 2020 and recovering to 11.4 tons in 2023. After a low of 0.4 tons in 2022, manufacture in Brazil rebounded to 7.8 tons in 2023. Globally, more than 99 per cent of the manufacture of diazepam in 2023 was reported by four countries: India, Italy, China and Brazil. Total manufacturers' stocks across all countries and territories declined slightly, dropping from 42.9 tons in 2022 to 40.3 tons in 2023. The countries with the largest stocks of diazepam in 2023 were China (10.4 tons), Italy (8.3 tons), Brazil (6.2 tons) and Denmark (3.7 tons).

58. Diazepam was also the most widely traded internationally controlled psychotropic substance in 2023, with 164 countries and territories reporting imports of the substance. Global imports of diazepam had increased steadily, from 32.5 tons in 2017 to a peak of 66.4 tons in 2021. However, imports then followed a downward trend, declining to 44.4 tons in 2022 and to 37.2 tons in 2023. The number of countries and territories importing

Figure 11. Benzodiazepines with significant presence on the licit market: shares of global manufacture by substance, based on gross weight, 2023

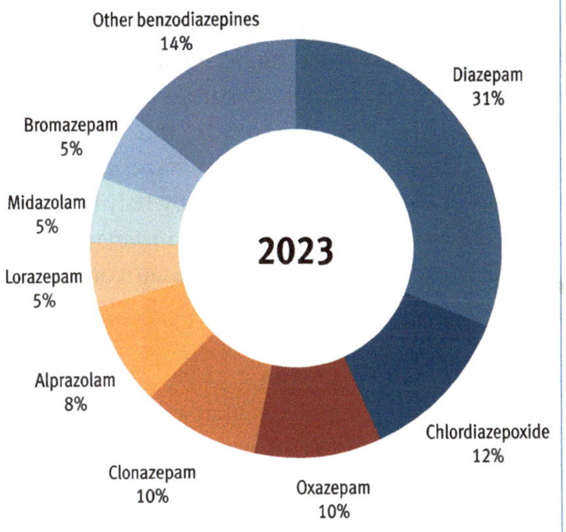

Figure 12. Diazepam: number of countries and territories reporting consumption, by region, 2019–2023

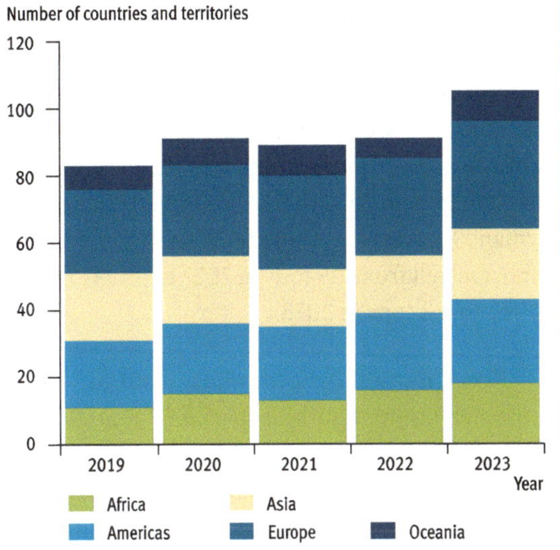

diazepam peaked at 176 in 2018 and then fluctuated in the years that followed. As noted above, 164 countries and territories reported imports of the substance in 2023, up from 160 in 2022. Imports of more than 1 ton in 2023 were reported by Ghana, Spain, the United States, the Democratic Republic of the Congo, Czechia, Germany, France, Bangladesh, Japan and Serbia (in descending order by quantity imported), which together accounted for approximately 60 per cent of total global imports. The main exporting countries in 2023 were Italy (16.3 tons), India (10.2 tons), Denmark (2.7 tons), Czechia (2.2 tons), Germany (1.8 tons), China (1.7 tons), Switzerland (1.1 tons) and Spain (0.7 tons). Taken together, those countries accounted for 93 per cent of global exports of the substance.

59. Among those countries and territories that provided data, the number that reported consumption data for diazepam increased significantly, from 91 in 2022 to 105 in 2023 (see figure 12). Cabo Verde reported the highest level of consumption of diazepam in 2023, at 20.90 $\text{S-DDD}_{\text{ptpd}}$, a significant increase from 5.74 $\text{S-DDD}_{\text{ptpd}}$ in 2022. Montenegro (14.37 $\text{S-DDD}_{\text{ptpd}}$), Portugal (13.88 $\text{S-DDD}_{\text{ptpd}}$) and Spain (13.68 $\text{S-DDD}_{\text{ptpd}}$) were among the other countries that reported consumption levels exceeding 10 $\text{S-DDD}_{\text{ptpd}}$ in 2023. Brazil also saw a sharp rise in consumption, reaching 12.03 $\text{S-DDD}_{\text{ptpd}}$ in 2023, compared with 1.41 $\text{S-DDD}_{\text{ptpd}}$ in 2022. Bosnia and Herzegovina reported a consumption level of 10.71 $\text{S-DDD}_{\text{ptpd}}$ in 2023, while Guyana reported 9.30 $\text{S-DDD}_{\text{ptpd}}$.

Midazolam

60. The manufacture of midazolam reached a record high of 25 tons in 2021, as demand for the substance increased owing to its use as a sedative for patients admitted to intensive care units with the coronavirus disease (COVID-19), as well as to its inclusion in the World Health Organization Model List of Essential Medicines. Manufacture dropped sharply in 2022, to 13.5 tons, and further to 9.2 tons in 2023, although it remained well above pre-2021 levels. Since 2016, more than 98 per cent of the global supply of midazolam has been manufactured in five countries, namely, Brazil, China, India, Israel and Italy. Brazil reported a significant increase in manufacturing, from 1.4 tons in 2022 to 3.1 tons in 2023. Manufacture in India continued to decline, dropping from 4.4 tons in 2022 to 2.9 tons in 2023. Italy also recorded a decrease, manufacturing 2.3 tons in 2023, down from 4.4 tons in 2022. Israel, a major manufacturer in previous years, did not report any manufacture in 2023. China manufactured 0.8 tons, an increase from 0.7 tons in 2022. Global manufacturers' stocks of midazolam came to 8.4 tons in 2023, down from 14.4 tons in 2022. The largest stocks were held by Brazil (1.8 tons), Italy (1.1 tons), France (1.0 tons), India (0.9 tons) and the United States (0.9 tons). The decline in global manufacturers' stocks of midazolam from 14.4 tons in 2022 to 8.4 tons in 2023 is primarily attributed to significant reductions in stock levels in Brazil (from 4.5 tons to 1.8 tons) and India (from 1.4 tons to 0.9 tons), among other countries.

61. From 2014 to 2023, the overall volume of midazolam imports reported worldwide averaged 10.7 tons per year. While the number of countries and territories reporting imports has remained relatively stable, the volume has increased significantly, reaching a 10-year high of 18.2 tons in 2021, driven by demand related to the COVID-19 pandemic. In 2022, imports decreased to 12.6 tons, followed by a further drop to 8.6 tons reported by a total of 159 countries and territories in 2023. The largest importer of midazolam in 2023 was Germany (2.9 tons); the other reporting countries and territories showed significantly lower import quantities. The overall decline in imports was primarily due to substantial reductions by major importers from previous years, such as Brazil, which imported just 0.2 tons, compared with 2.5 tons in 2022, and Türkiye, which reported a drastic decrease from 1.2 tons in 2022 to only 80 kg in 2023. Similarly, global exports of midazolam dropped from 20.9 tons in 2021 to 12.6 tons in 2022 and further to 9.1 tons in 2023. Exports were led by Italy (3.5 tons), Germany (2 tons) and India (1.2 tons), while other key exporters saw notable decreases. For instance, exports from Israel fell from 1.9 tons in 2022 to just 471 kg in 2023. Similarly, exports from India decreased from 2.8 tons in 2022 to 1.2 tons in 2023.

62. Consumption data on midazolam for 2023 were provided by 100 countries and territories. Greece (4.01 S-DDD_{ptpd}), Sint Maarten (3.97 S-DDD_{ptpd}), Brazil (3.18 S-DDD_{ptpd}) and Uruguay (2.30 S-DDD_{ptpd}) reported the highest rates of midazolam consumption. However, many countries and territories saw significant declines in consumption compared with previous years. Greece, despite leading the list, recorded a decrease from 7.08 S-DDD_{ptpd} in 2022. Similarly, consumption reported by Türkiye, which had surged to 2.34 S-DDD_{ptpd} in 2022, dropped to just 0.03 S-DDD_{ptpd} in 2023. Israel also saw a decline, from 1.41 S-DDD_{ptpd} in 2022 to 0.29 S-DDD_{ptpd} in 2023.

Clonazepam

63. Clonazepam, the only anti-epileptic benzodiazepine under international control, is also used for the treatment of panic disorders and anxiety. In 2023, global clonazepam manufacture reached a record high. After rising to 17.2 tons in 2021, followed by a decline to 10.7 tons in 2022, total manufacture surged to 17.9 tons in 2023. India was the largest manufacturer, reporting 11.4 tons in 2023, more than double the 5.2 tons reported in 2022. Brazil followed with 3.6 tons, up from 2.1 tons in 2022. Other significant manufacturers included Italy (1.6 tons) and China (1.04 tons). Switzerland, which had manufactured notable quantities in earlier years, reported only 3.7 kg in 2022 and did not report any manufacture of the substance in 2023. Stocks of clonazepam decreased slightly, from 6.6 tons in 2022 to 6.4 tons in 2023. Stocks in Switzerland dropped from 1 ton in 2022 to 472 kg in 2023. Mexico, which had 1 ton of stocks in 2022, reported no stocks in 2023. At the same time, Brazil saw an increase from 1.7 tons to 2.3 tons, making it the largest holder of clonazepam stocks in 2023. Stocks in Italy also decreased, falling from 900 kg in 2022 to 597 kg in 2023.

64. Global imports of clonazepam increased steadily until 2022, when they reached a record high of 15.1 tons. In 2023, however, imports declined to 11.4 tons, largely owing to significantly reduced imports by Germany (1.2 tons, compared with 6.8 tons in 2022) and Switzerland (870 kg, compared with 1.2 tons in 2022). In contrast, the United States (1.2 tons) and Brazil (960 kg) reported higher levels of imports compared with previous years. Spain reported no significant change, with imports of 1.1 tons in 2023, compared with 1.2 tons in 2022.

65. In 2023, 89 countries and territories reported consumption data for clonazepam, an increase from 78 in 2022. Brazil (12.79 S-DDD_{ptpd}) reported the highest consumption, showing a significant increase from 6.53 S-DDD_{ptpd} in 2022. Mexico saw the most substantial increase, as consumption rose from 0.28 S-DDD_{ptpd} in 2022 to 9.30 S-DDD_{ptpd} in 2023. Uruguay (8.05 S-DDD_{ptpd}), despite a decline from 14.08 S-DDD_{ptpd}, remained among the countries with the highest reported consumption. Consumption in Chile rose from 3.07 S-DDD_{ptpd} to 7.77 S-DDD_{ptpd}. Between 2022 and 2023, Costa Rica also reported a rise in consumption, from 4.89 S-DDD_{ptpd} to 7.22 S-DDD_{ptpd}, while Spain reported a decrease from 8.12 S-DDD_{ptpd} to 3.73 S-DDD_{ptpd}, and Portugal showed an increase from 2.38 S-DDD_{ptpd} to 5.90 S-DDD_{ptpd}.

Alprazolam

66. Alprazolam, a short-acting tranquillizer used in the short-term management of anxiety disorders, is one of the most frequently prescribed benzodiazepines worldwide. In 2023, global manufacture of the substance

reached a record high of 15.6 tons, up from 12.8 tons in 2022. India increased its manufacture significantly, from 6.9 tons in 2022 to 10.8 tons in 2023. The United States reported a decline in manufacture from 2.7 tons in 2022 to 2.1 tons in 2023. Italy reported total manufacture of 1.7 tons, China 513 kg and Australia 201 kg, with smaller quantities reported by a few other countries. Total global stocks of alprazolam dropped slightly, from 7.8 tons in 2022 to 7.4 tons in 2023, with the United States (2.3 tons), Italy (1.2 tons), India (797 kg) and China (745 kg) holding the largest quantities.

67. The total volume of alprazolam imported globally saw a sharp increase in 2023, reaching 14.9 tons, up from 10.1 tons in 2022. A total of 139 countries and territories reported imports in 2023. Israel saw a significant rise in imports, reaching 5.2 tons, a considerable increase from the 8 kg reported in 2022, making it the largest importer in 2023. The United States followed with 1.5 tons, showing a slight increase from 1.3 tons in 2022. Italy also reported an increase, importing 1.3 tons, up from 664 kg in 2022. Brazil imported 820 kg, down from 1.39 tons in 2022. Switzerland and Ireland also saw declines, with imports totalling 504 kg and 399 kg, respectively. Smaller quantities were imported by various other countries.

68. In 2023, a total of 85 countries and territories reported consumption data for alprazolam. Of the countries and territories that reported consumption, 11 reported rates of consumption of 10 S-DDD$_{ptpd}$ or higher and 26 reported rates below 10 S-DDD$_{ptpd}$ but higher than 2 S-DDD$_{ptpd}$. Among those countries and territories, Hungary (51.02 S-DDD$_{ptpd}$), Australia (29.54 S-DDD$_{ptpd}$), Portugal (26.23 S-DDD$_{ptpd}$), Spain (21.24 S-DDD$_{ptpd}$) and Montenegro (20.73 S-DDD$_{ptpd}$) were the top five consumers of the substance in 2023.

Lorazepam

69. The global manufacture of lorazepam increased from 8.6 tons in 2022 to 10.2 tons in 2023. That growth was primarily driven by India, where manufacture surged from 1.8 tons in 2022 to 3.1 tons in 2023, and by Germany, which saw a notable increase from 954 kg in 2022 to 2.3 tons in 2023. In contrast, Italy, while remaining the largest manufacturer, reported a decline from 5.4 tons in 2022 to 4.3 tons in 2023. Smaller quantities were manufactured in China, Costa Rica and the United States. Manufacturers' stocks increased from 6.9 tons in 2022 to 8.8 tons in 2023. Germany was the largest holder of stocks, with 2.6 tons, followed by Italy (1 ton), the Kingdom of the Netherlands (987 kg) and Canada (911 kg). Smaller quantities were held by 35 other countries.

70. In 2023, global imports of lorazepam reached a new low of 8.5 tons, continuing their downward trend from 8.6 tons in 2022 and 11.5 tons in 2020. Spain was the largest importer in 2023, at 1.2 tons, followed by the United States (1.2 tons), Ireland (741 kg), Canada (686 kg) and Germany (657 kg). Global exports of lorazepam followed a similar pattern, reaching 9 tons in 2023, down from 9.6 tons in 2022. In 2023, exports of lorazepam were again led by Italy, which exported 4.5 tons. Germany and India were also major exporters, exporting 1.6 tons and 1.3 tons, respectively. Those three countries were the only ones to export more than 1 ton of lorazepam in 2023.

71. Consumption of lorazepam was reported by 81 countries and territories in 2023, up from 70 in 2022. As in previous years, Portugal reported the highest level of lorazepam consumption, at 34.82 S-DDD$_{ptpd}$, followed by Spain (26.92 S-DDD$_{ptpd}$), Montenegro (14.13 S-DDD$_{ptpd}$), Belgium (12.92 S-DDD$_{ptpd}$) and Malta (11.98 S-DDD$_{ptpd}$). In addition, 21 other countries reported consumption levels between 2 and 10 S-DDD$_{ptpd}$. The remaining countries and territories reported consumption levels below 2 S-DDD$_{ptpd}$.

Bromazepam

72. The manufacture of bromazepam peaked at 15.2 tons in 2022 before dropping to 9.0 tons in 2023, returning to levels more typically observed in past years. The peak in 2022 was driven by Switzerland, which reported 5.9 tons after not reporting any manufacture in 2021. In 2023, Switzerland again reported no manufacture. Italy remained the largest manufacturer in 2023, at 6.2 tons. The other major manufacturers were India (1.7 tons) and Brazil (1.1 tons). In 2023, global stocks of bromazepam decreased to 8.8 tons, following a peak of 11.6 tons in 2022. Switzerland reduced its stocks significantly, from 5.5 tons in 2022 to 1.7 tons in 2023. Italy increased its stocks from 1.7 tons in 2022 to 2.5 tons in 2023, while France saw a decrease from 1.5 tons to 1.2 tons. Brazil maintained relatively stable stock levels, reporting 1.2 tons, a slight decrease from the 1.3 tons reported in 2022.

73. In 2023, global imports of bromazepam increased to 15.9 tons, up from 13.1 tons in 2022, driven by a significant rise in imports by Germany, which more than doubled, from 1.9 tons in 2022 to 4.5 tons in 2023. Serbia, on the other hand, saw a decrease in imports from 1.2 tons to 893 kg. Other key importers in 2023 included Pakistan (1.7 tons), France (1.6 tons) and Italy (837 kg). Total exports of bromazepam increased from 13.7 tons in 2022 to 16.3 tons in 2023. The main exporters in 2023 were Italy (5.8 tons), Switzerland (4.4 tons), Germany (3.2 tons) and India (1.7 tons).

74. The highest consumers of bromazepam in 2023 were Montenegro (15.47 S-DDD_{ptpd}) and Bosnia and Herzegovina (15.38 S-DDD_{ptpd}). The other countries reporting consumption levels above 4 S-DDD_{ptpd} for the year were France, with 5.43 S-DDD_{ptpd}, and Lithuania, where consumption remained steady at 4.75 S-DDD_{ptpd}.

Clobazam

75. Global manufacture of clobazam decreased to 8.7 tons in 2023 from 12.3 tons in 2022. This decline was primarily due to the absence of any reported manufacture by France, which had reported 4.5 tons for the previous year. In 2023, India led global manufacture with 6.6 tons, followed by Germany with 1.9 tons. Italy, Peru and the United States reported far smaller quantities.

76. Global imports of clobazam decreased slightly, to 7.4 tons in 2023, after relatively stable levels of 7.5 tons in 2022 and 7.9 tons in 2021. India was the largest importer of clobazam in 2023, with 1.2 tons, followed by France (999 kg), the United States (792 kg), Brazil (766 kg) and Indonesia (447 kg). Global exports were also largely unchanged from their 2022 level, amounting to 8.2 tons in 2023. France (3.4 tons), India (2.5 tons) and Germany (1.5 tons) were the only major exporters of clobazam in 2023.

77. Consumption of clobazam was reported by 66 countries and territories in 2023, up from 55 in 2022. Portugal and New Zealand exhibited the highest rates, reporting 1.11 S-DDD_{ptpd} and 1.10 S-DDD_{ptpd}, respectively. Uruguay followed at 0.89 S-DDD_{ptpd}, while Canada (0.83 S-DDD_{ptpd}) and France (0.73 S-DDD_{ptpd}) also recorded substantial consumption levels.

Chlordiazepoxide

78. The global manufacture of chlordiazepoxide has generally increased in recent years. After rising to 24.2 tons in 2021 and peaking at 25.5 tons in 2022, global manufacture decreased to 22.8 tons in 2023, mainly owing to reductions in Italy and India. Manufacture reported by Italy dropped from 13.6 tons in 2022 to 12.2 tons in 2023, and India reported a decrease from 11.3 tons to 9.6 tons. At the same time, the manufacture of chlordiazepoxide in China came to 978 kg in 2023, up from 600 kg in 2022. Manufacturers' stocks of chlordiazepoxide increased from 9.8 tons in 2022 to 10.7 tons in 2023 and were held in 31 countries, with the majority held in Italy (4.9 tons), India (1.4 tons), the United States (807 kg) and China (717 kg).

79. Global imports of chlordiazepoxide have fluctuated around 13 tons since 2020. After a peak of 14.1 tons in 2020, imports decreased to 13.9 tons in 2022 and 13 tons in 2023. Switzerland remained the largest importer of the substance in 2023, with 6.2 tons, followed by Pakistan and Egypt, both of which imported just over 1.2 tons each. Italy (12.4 tons), Switzerland (6.1 tons) and India (1.5 tons) accounted for more than 96 per cent of all exports of chlordiazepoxide in 2023.

80. Consumption of chlordiazepoxide was reported by 50 countries and territories in 2023. Iceland reported the highest level of consumption, at 1.29 S-DDD_{ptpd}, followed closely by Portugal with 1.20 S-DDD_{ptpd}. Other significant consumption levels were reported by Lebanon (0.76 S-DDD_{ptpd}), Chile (0.70 S-DDD_{ptpd}) and Albania (0.63 S-DDD_{ptpd}).

Oxazepam

81. The global manufacture of oxazepam has followed a downward trend since peaking at 27.5 tons in 2019. It decreased to 22.8 tons in 2020 and 22.7 tons in 2021, then continued its decline to 19.9 tons in 2022 and 18.8 tons in 2023. That downtrend can be attributed to decreased output in Italy, the leading manufacturer, where reported

manufacture dropped from 27.3 tons in 2019 to 15.3 tons in 2023. Manufacture in India, which has fluctuated in recent years, fell to 1.25 tons in 2023. At the same time, China, which had begun manufacturing significant quantities in 2021, reported 2.2 tons in 2023. Similarly, manufacturers' stocks of oxazepam have been declining since reaching a peak of 32.7 tons in 2020, dropping to 21.4 tons in 2022 and to 16.7 tons in 2023. Manufacturers' stocks of oxazepam were held in 24 countries, with the majority reported by France (7 tons), Italy (3.2 tons), Austria (995 kg) and Canada (931 kg) for 2023.

82. Global imports of oxazepam have declined since 2019, when they peaked at 30.5 tons. Imports dropped to 26.9 tons in 2020 and further to 19.9 tons in both 2022 and 2023. France was the largest importer of oxazepam, with 9.7 tons in 2023, up from 8.3 tons in 2022. Germany followed with 1.8 tons, showing a slight increase from 1.7 tons the previous year. Poland also increased its imports, to 1.6 tons, and South Africa imported 1.2 tons in 2023. Italy (16.4 tons), Germany (1.4 tons), Poland (979 kg) and India (959 kg) accounted for 97 per cent of all exports of oxazepam in 2023.

83. Consumption of oxazepam was reported by 34 countries in 2023. France reported the highest level of consumption of oxazepam, at 9.24 S-DDD_{ptpd}, followed by Iceland (5.63 S-DDD_{ptpd}), Norway (4.66 S-DDD_{ptpd}), Finland (4.38 S-DDD_{ptpd}), Austria (3.53 S-DDD_{ptpd}), the Kingdom of the Netherlands (3.30 S-DDD_{ptpd}), Portugal (2.29 S-DDD_{ptpd}), Sweden (2.16 S-DDD_{ptpd}) and Switzerland (2.01 S-DDD_{ptpd}).

English

Other benzodiazepines with a significant presence on the licit market

84. While alprazolam, bromazepam, chlordiazepoxide, clobazam, clonazepam, diazepam, lorazepam, midazolam and oxazepam comprise 90 per cent of the licit manufacture of benzodiazepines with a significant presence on the licit market, the remaining 10 per cent can be attributed to seven other substances, namely, nitrazepam, clorazepate, triazolam, temazepam, flunitrazepam, prazepam and flurazepam.

Nitrazepam

85. The manufacture of nitrazepam rose slightly, to approximately 2.9 tons in 2023, up from 2.7 tons the previous year. In 2023, Italy was the main manufacturer, with 1.5 tons, followed closely by India, which reported total manufacture of 1.4 tons. Stocks continued their downward trend, falling from 1.9 tons in 2022 to 1.4 tons in 2023. Italy held the largest stocks (292 kg) in 2023, followed by France (202 kg), with the remainder distributed among 22 other countries. Global imports of the substance increased to 2.0 tons in 2023, up from 1.5 tons in 2022. Similarly, exports rose from 1.6 tons to 2.0 tons. The consumption of nitrazepam was reported by 36 countries in 2023, with Malta reporting the highest consumption level (1.98 S-DDD_{ptpd}).

Clorazepate

86. The global manufacture of clorazepate, which had been in decline since 2019, showed a trend reversal in 2023, reaching 1.5 tons, up from 794 kg in 2022. Italy was the main manufacturer of the substance in 2023. Stocks of the substance saw a significant increase, from 1.5 tons in 2022 to 6.6 tons in 2023. Global imports of clorazepate also increased sharply, rising from 4.4 tons in 2022 to 8.3 tons in 2023. Global exports decreased slightly in 2023, with 4.2 tons exported globally. Consumption of clorazepate was reported by 25 countries in 2023, with Spain reporting the highest level of consumption at 3.97 S-DDD_{ptpd}.

Triazolam

87. After a spike in manufacture to 1.1 tons in 2021, the global manufacture of triazolam dropped to 252 kg in 2022 and further to 58 kg in 2023, marking the second lowest level since the substance was placed under international control. This decline was due to a significant decrease in manufacture in the United States and to the fact that no manufacture was reported by Italy. In 2023, three countries accounted for all manufacture of the substance: United States (31 kg), India (22 kg) and Republic of Korea (5 kg). Stocks were down by 75 kg and came to 308 kg in 2023; the United States (156 kg), Italy (72 kg) and Ireland (38 kg) held the majority. Imports

and exports of triazolam continued their downward trend in 2023. Imports decreased to 123 kg, and exports fell to the same level, marking a decline compared with 2022, when both came to approximately 170 kg. The consumption of triazolam was reported by 26 countries in 2023, with Austria reporting the highest level of consumption at 5.63 S-DDD_{ptpd}.

Temazepam

88. The manufacture of temazepam rebounded in 2023, rising to 6.9 tons from its lowest level in a decade, which was 5.4 tons in 2022. However, the total for 2023 remained well below the 11.6 tons reported in 2021. Italy was again the largest manufacturer of the substance in 2023, with manufacture rising to 6.3 tons. India followed with 181 kg, while Australia and Poland reported smaller quantities, namely, 200 kg and 131 kg, respectively. In 2023, stocks of temazepam dropped to 8.3 tons, continuing their downward trend from the previous years, with the majority held by Italy (2.5 tons) and by India and Canada, both of which reported about 1 ton. Total reported imports of temazepam increased slightly, from 7.7 tons in 2022 to 8.2 tons in 2023. Similarly, total exports increased to 8.5 tons in 2023, up from 7.5 tons in 2022. At 4.08 S-DDD_{ptpd}, the Kingdom of the Netherlands reported the highest level of consumption among the 19 countries that provided data.

Flunitrazepam

89. The manufacture of flunitrazepam has fluctuated significantly in recent years, dropping from 2.2 tons in 2020 to 36 kg in 2021, then rebounding to 182 kg in 2022 and to 544 kg in 2023. Italy led in the manufacture of the substance in 2023 with 240 kg, followed by Japan (165 kg) and India (138 kg). Stocks of flunitrazepam dropped to 614 kg in 2023, down from 979 kg in 2022, with Italy holding the largest quantity (193 kg). Imports of the substance fell from 1.8 tons in 2020 to 432 kg in 2022, but then rose to 809 kg in 2023. Similarly, global exports of the substance fell from 1.9 tons in 2020 to 530 kg in 2022 and rose to 945 kg in 2023. Uruguay reported the highest level of consumption of flunitrazepam in 2023, at 29.12 S-DDD_{ptpd}, nearly double the rate that it had reported in 2022. Nineteen other countries reported consumption of the substance.

Prazepam

90. The manufacture of prazepam rose significantly in 2023, reaching 3.9 tons, more than double the 1.7 tons reported in 2022, continuing the recovery from its low of 850 kg in 2020. Italy was the sole manufacturer of the substance in 2023. Stocks of prazepam increased to 3.4 tons in 2023, following a gradual decline from 7.1 tons in 2018 to 2.4 tons in 2022. Stocks were held by 12 countries. Imports of prazepam increased to 4 tons in 2023, up from 3.4 tons the previous year. Similarly, exports increased slightly, to 3.7 tons in 2023, compared with 3.5 tons in 2022. Only 13 countries reported consumption of prazepam in 2023, with the highest consumption reported by France (2.07 S-DDD_{ptpd}).

Flurazepam

91. Global manufacture of flurazepam rebounded to 2.8 tons in 2023 following a significant drop in 2022, when only 1.3 tons were manufactured, down from 3.4 tons in 2021. The increase was mostly due to a recovery in Italy, which reported 2 tons in 2023 after reporting manufacture of only 880 kg in 2022. Total stocks held in 2023 came to 2.3 tons, with Italy holding the largest amount (1 ton). Imports came to 1.7 tons in 2023, up from 1.5 tons in 2022. Similarly, exports increased to 2.1 tons in 2023, compared with 1.7 tons in 2022. Consumption was reported by 17 countries in 2023, with the highest consumption reported by Spain (0.92 S-DDD_{ptpd}).

Barbiturates

92. In 2023, only three internationally controlled barbiturates had a significant presence on the licit market (see table 10). The manufacture of pentobarbital and barbital increased, breaking the declining trend from the past decades. At the same time, the manufacture of phenobarbital continued its upward trend, increasing by almost 10 tons compared with the previous year. Amobarbital and butalbital, which are not listed in table 10, are still manufactured and traded in relatively large quantities.

Table 10. Barbiturates with significant presence on the licit market: total global manufacture and imports, ranked by number of importing countries and territories, 2023

Substance	*S-DDD (mg)*	*Manufacture (kg)*	*Imports (kg)*	*Number of importing countries and territories*
Phenobarbital	100	374 079.15	208 219.59	158
Pentobarbital	100	58 630.12	61 852.59	68
Barbital	500	58 313.31	2 965.38	22

Phenobarbital

93. In terms of gross weight, phenobarbital has been the most manufactured psychotropic substance under international control since 2012. In 2023, total reported manufacture of the substance came to 374 tons, up slightly from the 364.3 tons reported in 2022. Despite a decline of 46.8 tons from the previous year, China remained the largest manufacturer of phenobarbital, producing 174.9 tons in 2023. India, the other major manufacturer of the substance, reported a total of 130.9 tons in 2023, 31 tons more than in the previous year. Hungary (42.2 tons) and the Russian Federation (24.3 tons) were the only other countries to report any significant quantities manufactured in 2023.

94. Manufacturers' stocks of phenobarbital increased by 62.7 tons, from 182.4 tons in 2022 to 245.1 tons in 2023. The largest stocks were held by China (67.9 tons), followed by the Russian Federation (49.4 tons), Hungary (33.0 tons) and Brazil (26.0 tons). In addition, 12 countries reported stocks ranging from 1 to 10.8 tons, and another 33 countries reported stocks of less than 1 ton.

95. Imports of phenobarbital were reported by 158 countries and territories in 2023, making it one of the most widely traded psychotropic substances under international control. For 2023, the total volume of global imports came to 208.2 tons, reflecting a slight decrease from the 213 tons reported in 2022. Brazil reported the largest quantity of imports, at 41.2 tons, followed by the Russian Federation (23.0 tons), the United States (19.0 tons), Switzerland (10.0 tons) and Denmark (8.9 tons). Another 22 countries reported imports ranging from 1 to 6.8 tons. Imports reported by other countries and territories varied widely, from just a few dozen grams to several hundred kilograms.

96. Total exports of phenobarbital decreased significantly, from 226.8 tons in 2022 to 199.8 tons in 2023, in large part owing to a substantial reduction of exports from China, the second largest exporter in 2023. The country's phenobarbital exports fell from 86.1 tons in 2022 to 59.8 tons in 2023. The other leading exporters in 2023 were, in first place, India (79.0 tons), followed by Hungary (20.7 tons), Switzerland (9.7 tons), Denmark (9.1 tons), Germany (5.2 tons), Croatia (3.1 tons), France (2.7 tons), the Kingdom of the Netherlands (2.4 tons), Romania (2.3 tons) and Kenya (1.5 tons).

Figure 13. Phenobarbital: number of countries and territories reporting consumption, by region, 2019–2023

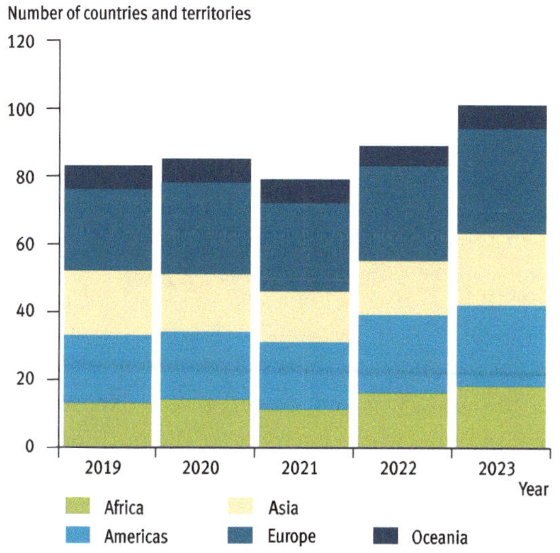

97. The number of countries and territories providing data on phenobarbital consumption increased from 89 in 2022 to 101 in 2023. A regional comparison of the number of countries and territories that provided consumption data from 2019 to 2023 is shown in figure 13. During that period, the Americas and Europe showed consistently high numbers of countries and territories providing data on phenobarbital consumption. In absolute terms, Oceania exhibited the lowest number of countries and territories providing such data each year. The number of countries and territories in Asia that provided data rose considerably in 2023, by five, while the corresponding number in Africa increased only slightly.

English

98. Among the countries and territories that provided data, Brazil reported the highest rate of phenobarbital consumption in 2023 (4.96 $S\text{-}DDD_{ptpd}$), a marginal increase from the previous year (4.95 $S\text{-}DDD_{ptpd}$). In Europe, San Marino (2.17 $S\text{-}DDD_{ptpd}$) was the highest consumer, followed by France (1.28 $S\text{-}DDD_{ptpd}$) and Montenegro (1.24 $S\text{-}DDD_{ptpd}$). In Africa, Seychelles reported the highest rate of consumption (4.81 $S\text{-}DDD_{ptpd}$), while Burkina Faso reported the lowest rate (0.01 $S\text{-}DDD_{ptpd}$). The intraregional disparity in the Americas was also wide; as noted above, Brazil (4.96 $S\text{-}DDD_{ptpd}$) reported the highest level of consumption in 2023, while Cuba reported the lowest (less than 0.03 $S\text{-}DDD_{ptpd}$). In Asia, the consumption levels among countries and territories that provided data also varied widely: China reported the highest rate of consumption (2.48 $S\text{-}DDD_{ptpd}$) and Iraq the lowest (0.003 $S\text{-}DDD_{ptpd}$). In Oceania, seven countries and territories provided data on the consumption of phenobarbital, with the highest rate of consumption reported by Australia (0.85 $S\text{-}DDD_{ptpd}$).

99. More detailed information regarding the consumption of phenobarbital can be found on the INCB website.

Pentobarbital

100. The United States and Germany were again the primary manufacturers of pentobarbital in 2023, reporting 33.6 tons and 24.6 tons manufactured, respectively. Japan reported a significant increase in its manufacture of the substance, which rose from 0.5 kg (2022) to 353 kg (2023). In total, 58.6 tons of pentobarbital were manufactured in 2023, a slight increase from the 56.0 tons reported in 2022. Manufacture in both Germany and the United States remained largely unchanged in 2023 compared with the previous year. India and Switzerland also reported manufacture of the substance, but in quantities of just a few grams each.

101. Manufacturers' stocks of pentobarbital rose from 43.0 tons in 2022 to 55.6 tons in 2023. The United States held approximately 16.8 tons of stocks, and Germany reported 16.7 tons, followed by the Kingdom of the Netherlands (8.0 tons), Denmark (3.4 tons), France (3.3 tons), Austria (2.4 tons), Switzerland and the United Kingdom (1.2 tons each). Sixteen other countries reported stocks, with each holding no more than a few hundred kilograms.

102. The Kingdom of the Netherlands led in imports of pentobarbital, reporting 16.5 tons for 2023, an increase of 4.7 tons from the 11.8 tons imported in 2022. Most of the country's imports were destined for re-export. Imports of pentobarbital reported by other countries were largely unchanged from previous years; the other main importers were Denmark (7.0 tons) and Germany (6.6 tons). Eight other countries reported imports of at least 1 ton. Another 18 countries reported imports between 100 kg and 1 ton, while the quantities reported by the remaining countries varied from a few grams to several dozen kilograms each.

103. Global exports of pentobarbital also increased to 47.5 tons in 2023, up from 41.5 tons in 2022. As a leading manufacturer of pentobarbital, Germany also led in exports of the substance, reporting 22.3 tons exported in 2023, slightly less than the 23.0 tons reported in 2022. The Kingdom of the Netherlands was the second largest exporter, at 11.8 tons, down slightly from the previous years. Denmark and Austria reported exports of more than 5.1 tons and 3.4 tons, respectively.

104. For 2022, a total of 44 countries and territories provided data on pentobarbital consumption, the same number as in 2021. Luxembourg reported the highest rate of consumption of the substance in 2023, at 4.12 $S\text{-}DDD_{ptpd}$, down slightly from 4.92 $S\text{-}DDD_{ptpd}$ in 2022. Denmark and Australia were the only other countries to report consumption exceeding 3 $S\text{-}DDD_{ptpd}$.

Barbital

105. The global manufacture of barbital increased from 48.6 tons in 2022 to 58.3 tons in 2023, surpassing the previous high of 57.9 tons reported for 2019. China remained the main manufacturer, reporting 36.8 tons manufactured in 2023, up from 30.6 tons in 2022. The only other countries to report the manufacture of barbital in 2023 were India (20.0 tons), Germany (1.1 tons) and Japan (341 kg). Manufacturing levels in those countries did not change significantly from the previous year, except in India, where the reported quantity increased from 13 tons to 20 tons. Manufacturers' stocks of barbital rose to 46.8 tons in 2023, a significant increase in comparison with the 29.1 tons reported for 2022. China held 40.7 tons of the substance, which represented nearly

87 per cent of global stocks and almost double the figure reported for 2022, while Germany (4.3 tons) and France (812 kg) held most of the remainder.

106. Trade in barbital was somewhat limited, with only 22 countries and territories reporting imports of the substance. Total imports for 2023 came to just under 3 tons, 234 kg above the 2.7 tons reported for 2022. The largest importer of barbital in 2023 was the United States (1.2 tons), followed by France (742.4 kg), Thailand (712.7 kg), Switzerland (166.8 kg) and the United Kingdom (97.5 kg). Total exports of the substance decreased by only 26 kg, to 2.6 tons in 2023, with Germany (1.9 tons) accounting for the largest share of global exports. Japan (357.6 kg) and Switzerland (187.5 kg) were the only other countries to report significant quantities exported.

107. With regard to the consumption of barbital, data are available from relatively few countries. For 2023, only 16 countries provided consumption data, and with the exception of China (0.06 $S\text{-}DDD_{ptpd}$), all of them reported consumption levels below 0.01 $S\text{-}DDD_{ptpd}$.

Other sedative-hypnotics

108. Of the eight sedative-hypnotics that are not benzodiazepines or barbiturates, only two are currently traded on the licit market: GHB and zolpidem. Conclusions based on the statistics regarding GHB should be drawn with care, as the S-DDD value for that substance is currently 7,500 mg, far higher than that of any other internationally controlled psychotropic substance. Given that most substances controlled under the 1971 Convention have S-DDD values ranging from 1 to 200 mg, the gross figures for GHB manufactured or traded may appear to suggest that it has a large market presence. In reality, the high S-DDD value for GHB arises from the fact that quantities of the substance must be manufactured at tens or even hundreds of times the amount of other psychotropic substances in order to reach equivalent dosage levels. This can be seen in table 11, in which the base weight of GHB for one defined daily dose for statistical purposes is 750 times that of zolpidem.

Table 11. Other sedative-hypnotics with significant presence on the licit market: total global manufacture and number of importing countries and territories, ranked by manufacture in S-DDD, 2023

Substance	*S-DDD (mg)*	*Manufacture (kg)*	*Manufacture (millions of S-DDD)*	*Number of importing countries and territories*
Zolpidem	10	40 740.39	4 074.04	118
Gamma-Hydroxybutyric acid	7 500	57 789.12	7.71	43

Gamma-Hydroxybutyric acid

109. Owing to its high S-DDD value, GHB must be manufactured in far larger quantities relative to other substances in order to meet global demand for medical and scientific purposes even though the substance is not as extensively traded as other psychotropic substances under international control.

110. For 2023, 57.8 tons of GHB were reported manufactured, representing a significant increase compared with the 51.9 tons reported for 2022. That increase was mainly due to the fact that Ireland reported no manufacture of the substance in 2021 but resumed manufacture in 2022 and 2023. Ireland (26.2 tons) was the leading manufacturer of GHB in 2023, followed by the United States (15.0 tons) and India (9.8 tons). Manufacturers' stocks of GHB increased drastically, from 119.7 tons in 2022 to 217.0 tons in 2023. The largest holder of stocks was Ireland, which reported just over 61.9 tons, followed by the United States (20.8 tons), France (6.5 tons), Ukraine (3.5 tons), Italy (3.0 tons) and Germany (2.8 tons). Switzerland reported a sharp decrease in its stocks of the substance, which fell from 2.5 tons in 2021 to 207.9 kg in 2023 owing to exports.

111. Imports of GHB were reported by 43 countries and territories in 2023 and totalled 62.9 tons, a significant decrease compared with the 78.1 tons reported by 41 countries in 2022. For 2023, the largest quantity of imports was reported by the United States (35.8 tons), followed by France (4.6 tons), Italy (4.1 tons), Belgium (4.0 tons), Latvia (2.7 tons), the Russian Federation (2.0 tons) and Spain (1.7 tons). Three other countries reported imports of GHB exceeding 1 ton, while the remaining countries and territories reported smaller quantities.

English

112. Exports of GHB came to 63.3 tons in 2023, down from 76.4 tons in 2022. The decline is attributable mostly to significant decreases in exports from Ireland, which saw exports decline from 42.5 tons in 2022 to 32.5 tons in 2023 but remained the leading exporter of the substance. Ireland was followed by the United States (7.1 tons), Germany (6.4 tons), India (4.1 tons), France (4.0 tons), Belgium (3.0 tons), Latvia (2.6 tons) and the United Kingdom (1.5 tons), and five other countries reported exports of GHB between 100 kg and 1 ton.

113. Consumption of GHB in 2023 was reported mainly by countries in Europe, as well as by Canada and the United States, continuing the trend from the past few years. The highest rate of consumption was reported by the United States (0.04 S-DDD$_{ptpd}$). Italy, Netherlands (Kingdom of the), Norway and Sweden each reported a consumption rate of 0.02 S-DDD$_{ptpd}$. Other countries that provided consumption data reported consumption levels below 0.02 S-DDD$_{ptpd}$.

Zolpidem

114. Zolpidem is one of the most widely traded psychotropic substances under international control. In 2023, 118 countries and territories reported imports of the substance, and consumption of zolpidem was reported in all regions of the world.

115. The manufacture of zolpidem rose slightly, from 39.1 tons in 2022 to 40.7 tons in 2023. As in past years, India was the primary manufacturer of the substance, reporting 25.8 tons manufactured in 2023, up 4.6 tons from 2022. Czechia reported the second largest quantity manufactured in 2023, at 7.6 tons, up from 0.4 tons in 2022. After reporting 4.2 tons in 2022, Brazil reported 3.1 tons manufactured in 2023. Japan (2.6 tons) and Argentina (1 ton) were also among the significant manufacturers of zolpidem in 2023. France, which had reported 3.5 tons in 2022, did not report any manufacture of the substance in 2023.

116. Global manufacturers' stocks of zolpidem nearly quintupled, rising from 18.4 tons in 2022 to 87.9 tons in 2023. The largest quantity was held by France (16.2 tons), followed by South Africa (6.7 tons), Brazil (4.4 tons), India (3.1 tons) and Czechia (3.0 tons). Smaller quantities were held by 33 other countries.

117. Total imports of zolpidem rose from 25.5 tons in 2022 to 35.8 tons in 2023. As in previous years, the United States reported the largest quantity of zolpidem imports, at 4.9 tons, down from 6.4 tons in 2022. Brazil (3.9 tons), Spain (3.0 tons), Germany (2.9 tons), Japan (1.6 tons), Poland (1.6 tons) and Argentina (1.5 tons) were the other main importers of the substance. Several of those countries imported zolpidem for the purpose of re-export.

118. Total exports of zolpidem have remained relatively steady for several years now. Exports totalling 37.6 tons were reported for 2023, a moderate decrease from the 41.6 tons exported in 2022, which itself had been an increase compared with the 37.3 tons reported for 2021. As the primary manufacturer of zolpidem, India was the leading exporter of the substance in 2023, at 13.6 tons, down from the 18.1 tons reported for 2022. Other major exporters were Czechia (7.7 tons) and France (5.4 tons). Germany, Netherlands (Kingdom of the), Serbia and Spain each reported exports of approximately 1 to 2 tons.

Figure 14. Zolpidem: number of countries and territories reporting consumption, by region, 2019–2023

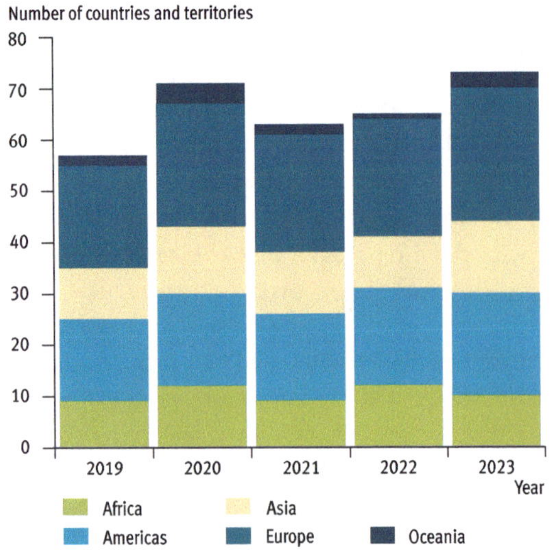

119. The total number of countries and territories providing data on zolpidem consumption in 2023 grew by 8, making for a total of 73 countries and territories (see figure 14). At the regional level, an increase in reporting was observed in all regions. Europe is the only region in which more than half of the countries and territories provided consumption data.

120. In 2023, Bosnia and Herzegovina reported the highest level of consumption of zolpidem worldwide, at 91.03 S-DDD$_{ptpd}$, followed by Czechia at 16.74 S-DDD$_{ptpd}$. Overall, among the countries

and territories that provided data, the average consumption of zolpidem in Europe was significantly higher than in other regions. In Africa, Morocco (0.54 S-DDD_{ptpd}) reported the highest level of consumption, while Angola (0.002 S-DDD_{ptpd}), reported the lowest. In the Americas, Brazil reported the highest consumption level (7.160 S-DDD_{ptpd}) and Ecuador the lowest (0.01 S-DDD_{ptpd}). In Asia, the Republic of Korea reported the highest consumption level (8.96 S-DDD_{ptpd}) and Maldives the lowest (0.04 S-DDD_{ptpd}). In Oceania, Australia reported the highest consumption level (0.97 S-DDD_{ptpd}), while the Federated States of Micronesia reported the lowest level (0.002 S-DDD_{ptpd}).

Meprobamate

121. Meprobamate, an anxiolytic listed in Schedule IV of the 1971 Convention, is the only non-benzodiazepine-type anxiolytic under international control that currently has any significant presence on the licit market. Although the substance is traded among only about a dozen countries, in terms of gross weight it is one of the most manufactured internationally controlled psychotropic substances.

Table 12. Meprobamate: total global manufacture, imports and number of importing countries, 2023

Substance	*S-DDD (mg)*	*Manufacture (kg)*	*Imports (kg)*	*Number of importing countries*
Meprobamate	1 200	39 535.67	49 194.72	14

122. Although the manufacture of and trade in the substance are limited to a small group of countries, the high dosage weight of meprobamate, like that of GHB, requires significant quantities of the substance to be manufactured in order to meet demand. As shown in table 12, 39.5 tons of meprobamate were manufactured in 2023, representing a significant decrease from the 97.1 tons reported in 2022. As in previous years, China and India were the largest manufacturers of the substance in 2023, reporting 26.0 tons and 13.5 tons manufactured, respectively. Global manufacturers' stocks of meprobamate came to 49.2 tons in 2023, representing a substantial increase from the value reported for 2022 (37 tons). China held the largest stocks (40.6 tons), followed by South Africa (3.8 tons). India and Lebanon also held significant stocks of the substance in 2023, with 1.9 tons and 1.2 tons, respectively.

123. Total imports of meprobamate came to 49.2 tons in 2023, up 4.4 tons from the 44.8 tons reported for 2022. South Africa accounted for more than half of all imports of the substance (26.4 tons), followed by India (15.8 tons) and the Democratic Republic of the Congo (3.8 tons). Exports of meprobamate fell from 114.4 tons in 2022 to 41.0 tons in 2023. As the main manufacturers of the substance, India and China also led in exports, with totals of 21.7 tons and 17.7 tons, respectively.

124. As the manufacture of and trade in meprobamate are limited to a small group of countries, consumption of the substance has also been very limited. In 2023, only 3 countries provided data regarding consumption of the substance, down from 13 in 2022. The highest level of consumption in 2023 was reported by Lebanon, at 0.21 S-DDD_{ptpd}, followed by Belgium (0.02 S-DDD_{ptpd}) and India (0.01 S-DDD_{ptpd}).

Buprenorphine

125. Of the three analgesics listed in Schedule III of the 1971 Convention, only one substance, buprenorphine, had a significant presence on the licit market in 2023. An opioid used mainly as an analgesic and in the treatment of opioid dependence, the substance was imported by 97 countries and territories in 2023 (see table 13).

Table 13. Buprenorphine: total global manufacture, imports and number of importing countries and territories, 2023

Substance	*S-DDD (mg)*	*Manufacture (kg)*	*Imports (kg)*	*Number of importing countries and territories*
Buprenorphine	8	15 537.57	9 915.08	97

English

126. The global manufacture of buprenorphine started to increase gradually in the late 1990s as the substance began to be used in higher doses for the treatment of pain and opioid addiction. After a significant decline in 2010, the reported global manufacture of the substance rose steadily, reaching 17.2 tons in 2018, but then decreased to 10.5 tons in 2019 because no manufacture was reported by the United Kingdom, the leading manufacturer of the substance up to that time. In 2023, total manufacture reached 15.5 tons, with four countries manufacturing significant quantities of the substance, namely, the United Kingdom (5.9 tons), Germany (2.6 tons), the United States (2.6 tons) and India (2.2 tons).

127. Trade in buprenorphine declined from 13.5 tons of imports in 2022 to 9.9 tons in 2023. As noted above, imports were reported by 97 countries and territories worldwide, led by the United States (6.6 tons), followed by France (642.2 kg), Germany (484.4 kg), the United Kingdom (272.6 kg) and Canada (246.9 kg). Three other countries imported approximately 100 kg each. As for exports, the United Kingdom (5.3 tons), Germany (1.6 tons) and Czechia (1.3 tons) were the primary exporters in 2023.

128. For 2023, 64 countries and territories provided data on the consumption of buprenorphine. Consumption was reported mostly in Europe and North America, as in previous years (see table 14). The highest rate of consumption for 2023 was reported by the United States (8.84 $S\text{-}DDD_{ptpd}$), followed by Iceland (3.60 $S\text{-}DDD_{ptpd}$), the United Kingdom (2.45 $S\text{-}DDD_{ptpd}$), Finland (2.25 $S\text{-}DDD_{ptpd}$) and Australia and Montenegro (both 2.11 $S\text{-}DDD_{ptpd}$). Australia reported the consumption of buprenorphine for the first time in 2023.

Table 14. Buprenorphine: rates of consumption in selected countries and territories, ranked by rate of consumption, 2021–2023

	S-DDD per 1,000 inhabitants per day		
Country or territory	*2021*	*2022*	*2023*
United States	9.17	9.16	8.84
Iceland	1.52	9.53	3.60
United Kingdom	3.30	2.13	2.45
Finland	2.05	2.10	2.25
Australia	–	–	2.11
Montenegro	2.21	2.10	2.11
Canada	1.92	2.01	2.10
Norway	–	1.98	1.97
Portugal	0.47	1.48	1.69
Sweden	1.55	1.59	1.64
France	–	–	1.48
Gibraltar	0.16	0.11	1.43
Austria	1.26	1.25	1.22
Germany	1.26	1.66	1.01
Poland	0.72	0.70	0.90

Exempted preparations

129. The reporting obligations under article 16 of the 1971 Convention require that parties report quantities of psychotropic substances used for the manufacture of other psychotropic substances, of exempt preparations and of non-psychotropic substances. These uses of psychotropic substances are distinct from the reported consumption of quantities used for medical and scientific purposes.

130. Article 3 of the 1971 Convention permits countries to exempt preparations containing psychotropic substances from some measures of control. Only preparations containing substances included in Schedules II, III or IV of the Convention can be exempted. Such exemptions can allow a country to make certain medicines more readily available in its territory or more easily traded.

131. Five substances included in Schedule II were used in quantities of 0.01 kg or more to manufacture exempted preparations in 2023 (see table 15). No use of levomethamphetamine was reported. In previous years, the United States had accounted for all of the levomethamphetamine used for exempted preparations. Germany accounted for all of the GHB used for the manufacture of exempted preparations in 2023, continuing the trend observed since 2019. Azerbaijan reported the use of metamfetamine to manufacture exempted preparations for the first time in 2023 and was the only country to do so. In 2023, Hungary reported the use of 1.38 tons of metamfetamine racemate. Australia accounted for almost all the *delta*-9-THC used for exempted preparations in 2023. In addition, the United States used less than 0.01 kg of dexamfetamine for exempted preparations.

Table 15. Schedule II substances used in the manufacture of exempted preparations, by quantity used, 2021–2023

Substance	*Quantity used (kg)*		
	2021	*2022*	*2023*
Metamfetamine racemate	0.03	127.49	1 388.89
Metamfetamine	0.05	0.01	412.00
Gamma-Hydroxybutyric acid	139.18	71.89	216.99
Delta-9-Tetrahydrocannabinol	8.96	25.51	8.85
Dexamfetamine	0.01	0.05	0.01
Methaqualone	<0.01	<0.01	<0.01
Methylphenidate	<0.01	–	<0.01
Phencyclidine (PCP)	<0.01	–	<0.01
Amfetamine	0.01	0.01	<0.01
Secobarbital	0.02	<0.01	–
3,4-Methylenedioxypyrovalerone (MDPV)	0.00	–	–
N-benzylpiperazine	–	0.01	–
CUMYL-PEGACLONE	5.41	–	–
Ethylone	–	<0.01	–
Levamfetamine	–	<0.01	–
Levomethamphetamine	178.02	247.25	–

132. The use of one substance listed in Schedule III in a quantity of 0.01 kg or more for the manufacture of exempted preparations was reported for 2023 (see table 16). Since 2017, the United States has been the only country to report the use of butalbital in the manufacture of exempted preparations. Most of the butalbital manufactured in the United States is used for the manufacture of such preparations, including codeine phosphate and acetaminophen, or for the manufacture of other non-psychotropic substances. The use of buprenorphine for exempted preparations has continued to decline since 2020, with only a negligible quantity used in 2022. In 2023, no use of buprenorphine for this purpose was reported.

Table 16. Schedule III substances used in the manufacture of exempted preparations, by quantity used, 2021–2023

Substance	*Quantity used (kg)*		
	2021	*2022*	*2023*
Butalbital	7 584.69	5 303.81	978.69
Buprenorphine	1.45	0.01	–
Pentobarbital	<0.01	<0.01	<0.01
Amobarbital	<0.01	–	<0.01

133. The use of 17 substances listed in Schedule IV of the 1971 Convention in quantities of 0.01 kg or more for the manufacture of exempted preparations was reported by 12 countries for 2023 (see table 17). Overall, the trends in the manufacture of exempted preparations have remained largely unchanged in the past few years. The

Russian Federation and Ukraine have accounted for the bulk of the phenobarbital used for exempted preparations. However, for 2022, Algeria for the first time reported the use of more than 1 ton of phenobarbital for such purposes. Germany accounted for most of the benzodiazepines shown in table 17 and for most of the zolpidem and oxazepam used in the manufacture of exempted preparations.

Table 17. Schedule IV substances used in the manufacture of exempted preparations, by quantity used, 2021–2023

	Quantity used (kg)		
Substance	*2021*	*2022*	*2023*
Phenobarbital	17 956.20	18 049.26	61 380.65
Diazepam	2 408.39	1 597.26	1 918.90
Zolpidem	1 897.51	1 790.10	1 811.52
Oxazepam	2 377.52	1 405.61	1 680.15
Barbital	1 615.36	1 531.50	1 001.14
Temazepam	410.04	594.15	516.09
Bromazepam	609.38	513.54	515.04
Prazepam	312.00	211.88	311.80
Chlordiazepoxide	93.96	218.54	197.60
Midazolam	277.62	228.28	183.37
Flurazepam	197.44	–	148.08
Lorazepam	224.94	85.69	94.44
Clonazepam	48.47	23.42	44.08
Alprazolam	32.69	43.47	33.72
Nitrazepam	59.03	18.00	26.00
Lormetazepam	37.66	3.63	11.43
Phentermine	8.21	0.01	0.01
Nordazepam	<0.01	<0.01	<0.01
Triazolam	–	–	<0.01
Flubromazolam	4.99	–	–

GLOBAL ASSESSMENT SYSTEM FOR PSYCHOTROPIC SUBSTANCES FOR MEDICAL AND SCIENTIFIC PURPOSES AND RECENT TRENDS

Assessment system for psychotropic substances and adherence by countries

Introduction

134. The drafters of the 1971 Convention did not include an estimates system for psychotropic substances similar to the one established for narcotic drugs controlled under the 1961 Convention as amended. It was only after the 1971 Convention entered into force that the international community determined that a global system was necessary so that countries could indicate their annual needs for psychotropic substances and prevent oversupply as well as the diversion of those substances from international trade.

135. In its resolutions 1981/7 and 1991/44, the Economic and Social Council invited countries to communicate to the Board from time to time their assessments of annual medical and scientific requirements for substances listed in Schedules II, III and IV of the 1971 Convention. Assessments are not required for substances included in Schedule I. Since the adoption of those resolutions, INCB has received such assessments from countries and territories and made them available to the international community by various means. The system has become a crucial pillar of the control of the international movement of psychotropic substances.

136. Since the adoption of the assessment system, the Board has advised countries that they should provide updated assessments of their annual licit requirements for psychotropic substances at least every three years. In addition, countries are invited to submit modifications of their assessments for specific substances as required, for example if their need for a substance exceeds a previously established assessment.

Submission of assessments and adherence to the assessment system for psychotropic substances

137. In general, countries and territories adhere to the assessment system for psychotropic substances even though the system was established outside the scope of the 1971 Convention and is entirely voluntary. All countries and territories recognized by the United Nations have established assessments for at least some substances controlled under the Convention. When a country has not established or is unable to establish its own assessments, the Board will do so to ensure that the most critical psychotropic substances can be imported by that country. In recent years, the only country for which the Board has had to establish assessments is South Sudan, in 2011.

138. Once established, assessments for psychotropic substances do not expire, and countries and territories therefore do not need to provide updated assessments for psychotropic substances on an annual basis, unlike for narcotic drugs controlled under the 1961 Convention as amended. It is recommended, however, that countries and territories update their assessments every three years in order to ensure that the assessments adequately reflect their medical and scientific needs. As a result, not all countries and territories submit new assessments each year, and if they believe their needs are being met, they may not modify any established assessments.

139. Each year, many countries and territories provide the Board with updated assessments for certain psychotropic substances. In the period 2014–2023, 90 to 104 countries and territories provided a total of 2,690 to 3,700 assessments for psychotropic substances each year (see table 18). During the same period, 88 to 104 countries and territories submitted a total of 369 to 675 modifications to their established assessments for psychotropic substances each year. During that 10-year period, a total of 206 countries and territories provided at least one assessment or modification to an established assessment for a psychotropic substance.

Table 18. Assessments for psychotropic substances and modifications received from countries and territories, 2014–2023

Year	*Assessments*	*Countries and territories submitting assessments*	*Modifications*	*Countries and territories submitting modifications*
2014	2 797	96	369	92
2015	2 690	92	513	98
2016	2 965	102	481	96
2017	3 192	104	398	88
2018	3 284	97	421	95
2019	3 700	97	500	90
2020	3 188	90	494	104
2021	2 983	94	607	90
2022	3 572	94	507	89
2023	3 680	94	675	94

140. The substances for which countries and territories provided the largest numbers of updated assessments or modifications of established assessments were also among the most actively manufactured and traded substances.

In total, 146 substances – nearly all of those included in Schedules II, III and IV of the 1971 Convention – were assessed or had an established assessment modified by at least one country or territory in the period 2014–2023. The substances for which the largest numbers of assessments or modifications were received for 2023 are shown in table 19.

Table 19. Psychotropic substances with the most assessments or modifications to assessments by countries and territories for 2023

Substance	*Assessments*	*Substance*	*Modifications*
Midazolam	100	Methylphenidate	42
Diazepam	100	Phenobarbital	23
Phenobarbital	99	Dexamfetamine	20
Clonazepam	95	Pentobarbital	18
Alprazolam	93	Buprenorphine	17

141. For 2025, 70 countries and territories have provided a total of 2,428 assessments for psychotropic substances. For those 144 countries and territories that have not provided updated assessments for 2025, their previously established assessments for 2024 will be carried over. Unlike in the estimates system for narcotic drugs, the reported stocks and consumption of psychotropic substances for one year do not affect assessments for those substances in the following year. The substances for which the largest numbers of countries and territories have updated their assessments for 2025 can be found in table 20.

Table 20. Psychotropic substances most assessed by countries and territories for 2025

Substance	*Assessments*
Diazepam	70
Midazolam	70
Clonazepam	68
Phenobarbital	67
Alprazolam	65

142. Assessments for 2025 for all countries and territories can be found in the online annexes. As countries and territories are able to update their assessments for psychotropic substances at any time, the most up-to-date assessments are available from the INCB website.

Trends in quantities of psychotropic substances assessed by countries and territories

143. As countries and territories are not required to update their assessments for psychotropic substances on an annual basis, global assessments for psychotropic substances do not tend to change significantly from one year to the next. Nonetheless, as indicated in the previous section, many countries regularly modify their global assessments in the course of the calendar year. The analysis below covers assessments as they stood at the end of 2023 and 2024 and for the beginning of 2025.

144. For 2025, the most assessed psychotropic substances by gross weight are phenobarbital (876.1 tons), GHB (238.0 tons), meprobamate (175.5 tons), methylphenidate (146.7 tons), diazepam (124.1 tons), pentobarbital (102.2 tons), zolpidem (92.8 tons), phentermine (62.2 tons), chlordiazepoxide (57.8 tons) and barbital (50.9 tons) (see figure 15). The assessments for phenobarbital for 2025 have decreased from 923.8 tons for 2024. Similarly, the assessments for meprobamate, diazepam and barbital have declined compared with previous years. Assessments of methylphenidate have increased by approximately 10 tons. In addition, assessments of phentermine for 2025 have almost doubled compared with those for 2023, largely driven by increased assessments by Mexico and the United States.

Figure 15. Most assessed psychotropic substances, based on gross weight, 2023–2025

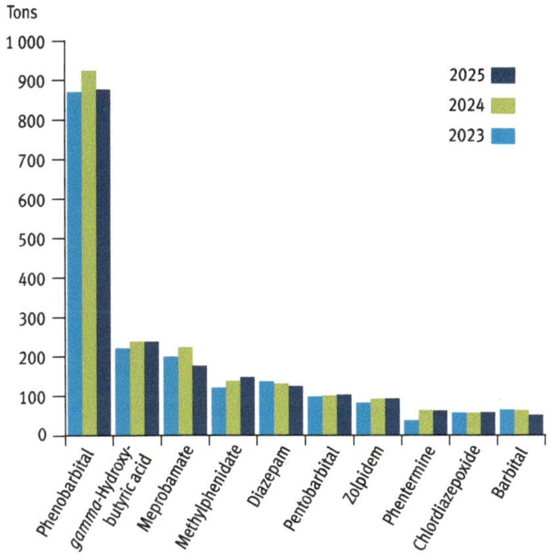

Figure 16. Most assessed psychotropic substances, based on S-DDD, 2023–2025

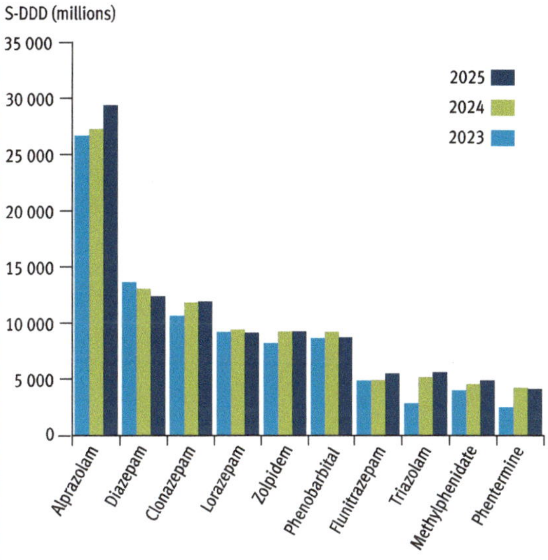

145. When considered in terms of dosage (S-DDD), the most assessed psychotropic substances are very different from those expressed in terms of gross weight. For 2025, the most assessed substances in terms of S-DDD are alprazolam (29.4 billion S-DDD), diazepam (12.4 billion S-DDD), clonazepam (11.9 billion S-DDD), lorazepam (9.2 billion S-DDD), zolpidem (9.3 billion S-DDD), phenobarbital (8.8 billion S-DDD), flunitrazepam (5.5 billion S-DDD), triazolam (5.6 billion S-DDD), methylphenidate (4.9 billion S-DDD) and phentermine (4.1 billion S-DDD).

146. As can be seen in figure 16, global assessments of alprazolam are more than double those of diazepam, the second most assessed substance. Notably, the assessments for alprazolam for 2025 have increased by 2.7 billion S-DDD compared with those for 2023. Similarly, assessments of triazolam for 2025 doubled compared with 2023. In terms of both gross weight and S-DDD, assessments for diazepam have declined. The other substances most assessed in terms of S-DDD exhibited only slight changes and fluctuations from 2023 to 2025.

English

OBSERVATIONS SUR LES STATISTIQUES ET LES PRÉVISIONS COMMUNIQUÉES SUR LES SUBSTANCES PSYCHOTROPES

Aperçu général

L'analyse contenue dans la présente partie de la publication technique sur les substances psychotropes fait fond sur les données statistiques et les données relatives aux prévisions communiquées par les gouvernements. Sa qualité dépend de celle des données communiquées.

La première section contient une présentation des principales tendances qui se dégagent des données communiquées par les pays et territoires, à commencer par un aperçu général de la situation concernant les 170 substances psychotropes qui étaient placées sous contrôle international en 2023, l'accent étant mis sur les grandes tendances déduites des données. On y trouvera des informations sur les faits nouveaux liés au contrôle de ces substances ainsi que sur les modifications apportées aux Tableaux de la Convention sur les substances psychotropes de 1971.

La première section se poursuit par une analyse détaillée des substances qui ont présenté le plus grand intérêt en 2023. L'analyse est ventilée par famille de drogues, à commencer par le tétrahydrocannabinol (THC) et le *delta*-9-THC, les hallucinogènes méthylènedioxy-3,4 méthamphétamine (MDMA), psilocybine et psilocine (psilotsine), suivis par les stimulants, les benzodiazépines, les barbituriques, les autres sédatifs-hypnotiques, les anxiolytiques (en particulier le méprobamate) et la buprénorphine. Les données les plus pertinentes concernant la fabrication, les importations, les exportations, les stocks et la consommation déclarée pour 2023 y sont examinées et les tendances qui en ressortent y sont comparées à celles des années précédentes. Des analyses et des informations supplémentaires sont fournies sur les substances utilisées dans la fabrication des préparations exemptées.

La deuxième section contient une analyse du système des prévisions relatives aux substances psychotropes et un examen des prévisions mondiales communiquées par les pays et territoires.

Toutes les données relatives à la consommation utilisées sont celles que les pays et territoires ont communiquées à l'Organe international de contrôle des stupéfiants (OICS) dans leurs rapports statistiques annuels. Sauf indication contraire, toutes les valeurs se rapportant à la consommation sont exprimées en doses quotidiennes déterminées à des fins statistiques (S-DDD) par millier d'habitants et par jour (S-DDD_{ptpd}). Cette unité de mesure a été adoptée par l'OICS pour mesurer la consommation de substances psychotropes, conformément à l'approche adoptée par le centre collaborateur de l'Organisation mondiale de la Santé pour une méthode d'établissement de statistiques sur les drogues.

L'analyse contenue dans la présente publication ne rend compte que des aspects les plus importants des activités licites concernant les substances psychotropes placées sous contrôle international. Les données complètes pour 2023, y compris les données sur la consommation, et les prévisions pour 2025, peuvent être consultées au format électronique sur le site Web de l'OICS.

TENDANCES RELATIVES AUX SUBSTANCES PSYCHOTROPES QUI SE DÉGAGENT DES DONNÉES COMMUNIQUÉES

Situation en ce qui concerne les substances psychotropes en 2023

1. Comme on le voit sur le tableau II de la présente publication, au 1er novembre 2024, 163 pays et 14 territoires avaient fourni leurs rapports statistiques annuels, comme cela est prévu à l'article 16 de la Convention sur les substances psychotropes de 1971. Ces chiffres sont en hausse par rapport à l'année précédente, au cours de laquelle 155 pays et 14 territoires avaient fourni leurs rapports statistiques annuels avant le 1er novembre.

2. Les performances en matière de communication de données se sont améliorées dans toutes les régions en 2023 par rapport à 2022. Pour 2023, au moins 68 % de l'ensemble des pays et territoires de chaque région ont fourni le rapport statistique annuel demandé (voir tableau 1).

Tableau 1. Statistiques annuelles sur les performances en matière de communication des données des pays et territoires, par région (2022 et 2023)

	Nombre de pays et territoires	
Région	*2022*	*2023*
Afrique	39 sur 57 (68 %)	42 sur 57 (74 %)
Amériques	36 sur 45 (80 %)	37 sur 45 (82 %)
Asie	40 sur 48 (83 %)	41 sur 48 (85 %)
Europe	41 sur 43 (95 %)	42 sur 43 (98 %)
Océanie	13 sur 22 (59 %)	15 sur 22 (68 %)

3. À la fin de 2023, 170 substances psychotropes étaient placées sous contrôle international, contre 167 à la fin de 2022. En mars 2023, la Commission des stupéfiants a décidé d'inscrire l'ADB-BUTINACA, l'*alpha*-PiHP et la 3-méthylméthcathinone au Tableau II de la Convention de 1971 et les substances sont passées sous contrôle international en novembre 2023.

4. Les substances psychotropes placées sous contrôle international comprennent plusieurs catégories et types de médicaments et sont utilisées pour traiter de très nombreux problèmes de santé. La plupart des substances psychotropes fabriquées et consommées sont des sédatifs-hypnotiques, des anxiolytiques et des antiépileptiques, y compris des barbituriques et des benzodiazépines. L'autre groupe important de substances fabriquées comprend les stimulants, principalement les amphétamines et le méthylphénidate. Les autres substances régulièrement fabriquées (hallucinogènes, analgésiques et antianémiques) ne représentent qu'une faible proportion de la quantité totale de substances psychotropes fabriquées.

5. Les tendances générales qui se dégagent de la fabrication de substances psychotropes placées sous contrôle international sont restées globalement les mêmes entre 2022 et 2023. En termes de poids brut, la substance la plus fabriquée dans le monde a été le phénobarbital, avec 374 tonnes, soit une quantité bien plus importante que pour n'importe quelle autre substance (voir fig. 1). Le méthylphénidate a été la deuxième substance la plus fabriquée dans le monde, avec 82,6 tonnes, ce qui, selon les données de l'Organe international de contrôle des stupéfiants (OICS), représente la plus grosse quantité de cette substance jamais fabriquée dans le monde en une seule année. La fabrication de méprobamate s'est classée au deuxième rang en 2022, mais a reculé de manière significative en 2023, la fabrication déclarée ayant chuté de plus de moitié pour s'établir à 39,5 tonnes.

6. Considérées en termes de doses (S-DDD), les substances psychotropes fabriquées en plus grosses quantités en 2023 ne sont pas les mêmes que si l'on se base sur le poids brut (voir fig. 2). En 2023, l'alprazolam était la substance la plus fabriquée, avec plus de 15,5 milliards de S-DDD, soit près du triple des 5,8 milliards de S-DDD déclarées pour le diazépam, qui était la deuxième substance la plus fabriquée. Les autres substances psychotropes

Figure 1. Substances psychotropes les plus fabriquées dans le monde, sur la base du poids brut (2023)

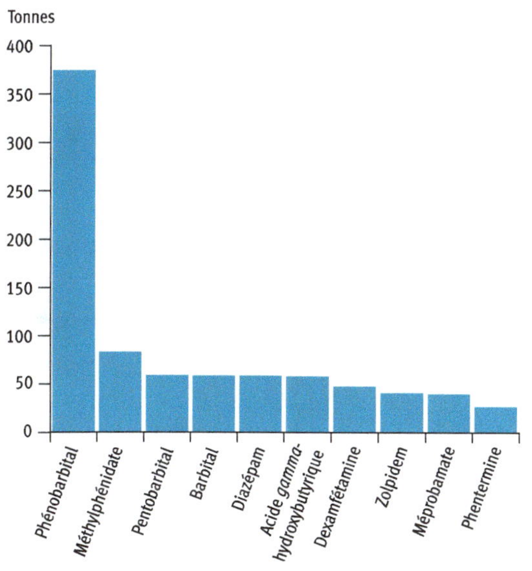

Figure 2. Substances psychotropes les plus fabriquées dans le monde, sur la base du nombre total de S-DDD (2023)

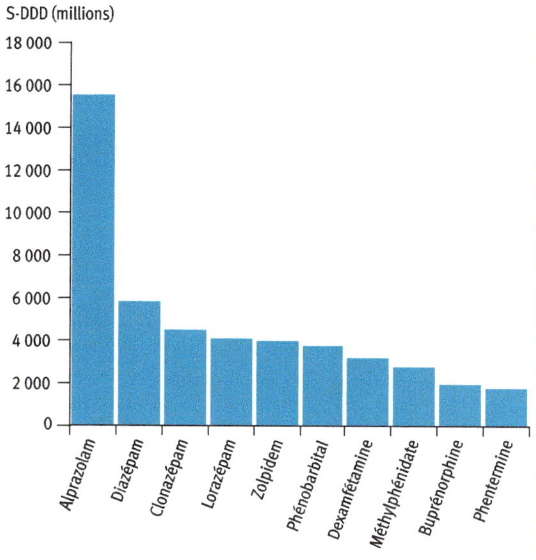

les plus fabriquées en 2023 en termes de doses étaient le clonazépam (4,48 milliards de S-DDD), le lorazépam (4,08 milliards de S-DDD), le zolpidem (3,97 milliards S-DDD), le phénobarbital (3,74 milliards S-DDD), la dexamfétamine (3,18 milliards S-DDD), le méthylphénidate (2,75 milliards S-DDD), la buprénorphine (1,94 milliard S-DDD) et la phentermine (1,77 milliard S-DDD). En 2023, 23 autres substances psychotropes ont été fabriquées en quantités supérieures à 100 millions de doses.

7. Les principaux pays producteurs de substances psychotropes sont généralement restés les mêmes que les années précédentes. En 2023, l'Inde était le plus grand fabricant en termes de poids brut car elle est le principal fabricant de plusieurs barbituriques et benzodiazépines. La Chine se plaçait au deuxième rang, principalement parce qu'elle est un important fabricant de plusieurs barbituriques. Les États-Unis d'Amérique, l'Italie et l'Allemagne complètent la liste des cinq premiers fabricants en termes de poids brut. En termes de S-DDD, les cinq premiers pays étaient les mêmes, si ce n'est que l'Italie est arrivée en deuxième position et la Chine en quatrième. La Suisse, par exemple, qui a toujours déclaré fabriquer des quantités beaucoup plus importantes de substances psychotropes (plus de 80 tonnes en 2018), en a déclaré beaucoup moins ces dernières années (7,4 tonnes en 2023), principalement en raison de l'arrêt de la fabrication d'acide *gamma*-hydroxybutyrique (GHB) et de *N*-benzylpipérazine (BZP).

8. En ce qui concerne le commerce international, six benzodiazépines figuraient parmi les substances psychotropes les plus échangées en 2023 (voir tableau 2). Le phénobarbital était le barbiturique placé sous contrôle international le plus échangé et le méthylphénidate le stimulant qui l'était le plus. Le sédatif non barbiturique le plus vendu qui ne soit pas de type benzodiazépine était le zolpidem. Le nombre de pays et territoires déclarant des importations de buprénorphine a continué d'augmenter par rapport aux années précédentes, bien que le volume des échanges ait été plus faible en 2023 qu'en 2022.

9. Comme les années précédentes, le diazépam a été la substance psychotrope placée sous contrôle international la plus largement importée en 2023, 164 pays et territoires en ayant déclaré des importations pour un total de 37,2 tonnes, soit la quantité la plus faible depuis 2017. Toujours en 2023, les importations totales de midazolam, de phénobarbital et de clonazépam étaient inférieures de 10 à 30 % à celles de 2022. En revanche, les importations d'alprazolam ont augmenté de près de 50 % sur la même période. Les volumes importés des autres substances les plus largement commercialisées n'ont pas connu de changements significatifs entre 2022 et 2023.

Figure 3. Substances psychotropes les plus consommées dans le monde, sur la base du nombre total de S-DDD (2023)

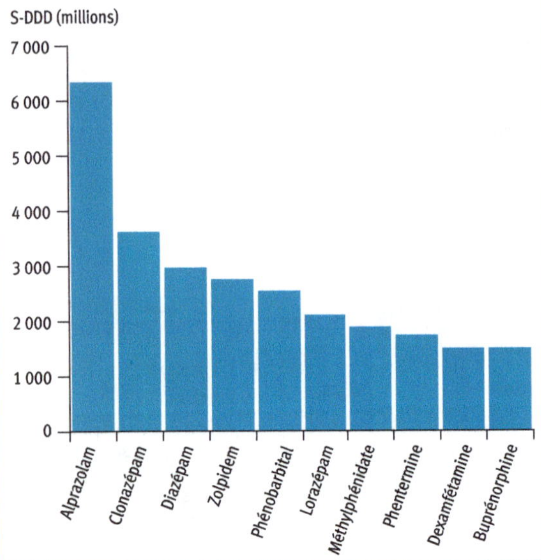

Figure 4. *Delta*-9-tétrahydrocannabinol : fabrication et stocks (2014-2023)

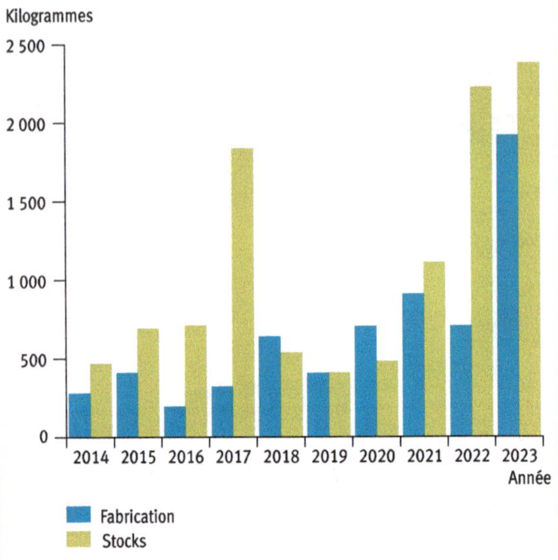

Tableau 2. Substances psychotropes placées sous contrôle international les plus largement commercialisées (2023)

Substance	*S-DDD (mg)*	*Total des importations (en kg)*	*Total des importations (en million de S-DDD)*	*Nombre de pays et territoires importateurs*
Diazépam	10	37 180,25	3 718,02	164
Midazolam	15	8 551,21	570,08	159
Phénobarbital	100	208 219,59	2 082,20	158
Clonazépam	4	11 374,47	2 843,62	142
Alprazolam	1	14 904,43	14 904,43	139
Lorazépam	2,5	8 540,29	3 416,12	126
Méthylphénidate	30	59 952,31	1 998,41	120
Zolpidem	10	35 814,82	3 581,48	118
Bromazépam	10	15 861,96	1 586,20	113
Buprénorphine	8	9 915,08	1 239,39	97

10. Au total, 111 pays et territoires (soit 63 % de ceux qui ont envoyé leurs statistiques annuelles) ont communiqué des données concernant la consommation d'au moins une substance psychotrope en 2023, alors qu'ils n'étaient que 100 en 2022. Les taux d'envoi de données relatives à la consommation ont varié considérablement d'une région à l'autre. Ainsi, en 2023, 20 pays et territoires d'Afrique (35 % du nombre total de pays et territoires de la région) en ont fourni, 25 pays et territoires des Amériques (56 % du nombre total de pays et territoires de la région), 22 pays et territoires d'Asie (46 % du nombre total de pays et territoires de la région), 35 pays et territoires d'Europe (81 % du nombre total de pays et territoires de la région) et 9 pays et territoires d'Océanie (41 % du nombre total de pays et territoires de la région).

11. Comme les valeurs exprimées en S-DDD établies pour les substances psychotropes peuvent varier considérablement d'une substance à l'autre (voir le tableau III de la présente publication), une analyse des données de consommation par poids brut ne refléterait pas fidèlement les tendances de la consommation mondiale. Les données relatives à la consommation exprimées en nombre total de S-DDD rendent mieux compte des schémas de consommation des pays et territoires déclarants et se prêtent mieux à l'analyse. La figure 3 présente les substances psychotropes les plus consommées dans le monde en 2023 en termes de nombre total de doses (S-DDD).

12. En 2023, l'alprazolam était la substance la plus consommée, avec plus de 6,3 milliards de S-DDD dans le monde, soit près de 1,5 milliard de plus qu'en 2022. La consommation de clonazépam a plus que doublé, passant de 1,6 milliard de S-DDD en 2022 à 3,6 milliards en 2023. La consommation de diazépam a également augmenté, passant d'environ 1 milliard de S-DDD à près de 3 milliards en 2023. La consommation des autres substances les

plus consommées en 2023 a connu des augmentations allant de 5 à 50 %. En revanche, la consommation mondiale d'estazolam a fortement diminué, passant de plus de 3,1 milliards de S-DDD en 2022 à 1,2 milliard en 2023.

Tétrahydrocannabinol et *delta*-9-tétrahydrocannabinol

13. Le tétrahydrocannabinol (THC) est un cannabinoïde présent naturellement dans la plante de cannabis, mais qui peut aussi être synthétisé chimiquement. Tous les isomères du THC sont inscrits au Tableau I de la convention de 1971, à l'exception de l'isomère *delta*-9-tétrahydrocannabinol (*delta*-9-THC), qui est inscrit au Tableau II. L'usage licite du THC et du *delta*-9-THC a été limité depuis qu'ils ont été placés sous contrôle international. Toutefois, l'activité licite liée à ces substances a augmenté ces dernières années, de plus en plus de pays ayant autorisé l'usage de certaines préparations de *delta*-9-THC à des fins médicales.

Tableau 3. Tétrahydrocannabinol et *delta*-9-tétrahydrocannabinol : fabrication licite et stocks au niveau mondial (total), 2023

Substance	*Quantité fabriquée (en kg)*	*Stocks (en kg)*
Tétrahydrocannabinol (Ensemble des isomères inscrits au Tableau I)	66,24	31,00
Delta-9-tétrahydrocannabinol	1 919,36	2 378,48

14. Comme on le voit sur le tableau 3, la fabrication de THC reste très limitée. Comme en 2022, c'est l'Australie (62,93 kg) qui a fabriqué la majeure partie de la quantité déclarée en 2023. Le commerce du THC est également très limité, seuls quelques pays déclarant des importations ou des exportations. Le Canada était le plus gros exportateur en 2023, avec 560,81 kg, tandis que les États-Unis étaient le plus gros importateur, avec 84,01 kg. L'activité de ces deux pays a constitué la quasi-totalité des échanges en 2023, seuls quelques autres pays ayant fait état de petites quantités importées ou exportées. L'Australie était le plus gros consommateur de THC en 2023, avec une consommation de 46,99 kg. Aucun autre pays ayant fourni des données sur la consommation de THC n'a fait état d'une consommation supérieure à quelques grammes[1].

15. En ce qui concerne le *delta*-9-THC, l'activité licite liée à cette substance s'est considérablement développée au cours des dernières années, de plus en plus de pays ayant autorisé l'utilisation de produits pharmaceutiques et d'autres préparations en contenant. Les quantités de *delta*-9-THC fabriquées ont varié depuis 2014, mais sont d'une manière générale en augmentation depuis 2020, année au cours de laquelle un total de 706,4 kg a été déclaré (voir fig. 4). En 2023, 1,92 tonne de *delta*-9-THC a été fabriquée dans le monde ; la plus grande quantité a été déclarée par le Royaume-Uni de Grande-Bretagne et d'Irlande du Nord (602,8 kg), suivi de l'Afrique du Sud (514,4 kg), de l'Allemagne (443,4 kg), de l'Australie (207,2 kg) et des États-Unis (139,4 kg).

ENCADRÉ 1. TÉTRAHYDROCANNABINOL ET *DELTA*-9-TÉTRAHYDROCANNABINOL : CHANGEMENTS DANS LA COMMUNICATION DES INFORMATIONS EN 2024

À partir de 2024, l'Organe international de contrôle des stupéfiants a conseillé aux gouvernements de revoir leurs procédures de communication d'informations au titre de la Convention unique sur les stupéfiants de 1961 telle que modifiée par le Protocole de 1972 et de la Convention sur les substances psychotropes de 1971, pour le cannabis et les cannabinoïdes dérivés par des procédés naturels et synthétiques.

L'OICS a recommandé aux pays et territoires de ne plus déclarer les quantités d'extraits ou de teintures de cannabis fabriquées, commercialisées, stockées, utilisées ou consommées au titre de la Convention de 1961 telle que modifiée, mais plutôt de déclarer toute préparation ou tout sous-produit obtenu à partir du cannabis en fonction des cannabinoïdes, notamment le tétrahydrocannabinol (THC) et le *delta*-9-THC, qu'il contient et qui sont placés sous contrôle en vertu de la Convention de 1971.

L'OICS a reconnu que la communication d'informations relatives au THC et au *delta*-9-THC peut être difficile pour certains pays et territoires en fonction de leurs systèmes de contrôle ou de collecte de données. La quantité d'isomères de THC fabriqués à partir de matières naturelles peut varier en fonction de la matière première et du processus d'extraction utilisé.

[1] La consommation de tétrahydrocannabinol (THC) ne peut être exprimée qu'en termes de poids brut, car aucune dose journalière définie à des fins statistiques (S-DDD) n'a été établie pour cette substance.

16. Les stocks de *delta*-9-THC détenus par les fabricants ont également varié de manière significative entre 2014 et 2023, et ils sont en nette augmentation depuis 2020, année au cours de laquelle ils s'établissaient à 481,9 kg. Ils sont passés à 1,11 tonne en 2021, puis à 2,22 tonnes en 2022. Pour 2023, les stocks des fabricants mondiaux s'élevaient à 2,38 tonnes. En 2023, c'est le Royaume-Uni qui détenait le stock le plus important (1,1 tonne), suivi de l'Afrique du Sud (426,5 kg), de l'Allemagne (398,4 kg), des États-Unis (313,1 kg) et de l'Australie (98,3 kg). Quatorze autres pays ont déclaré détenir des stocks de *delta*-9-THC, mais en très petites quantités.

17. Peu de pays font état d'une consommation de *delta*-9-THC, seuls sept pays ayant fourni des données pour 2023. Avant 2022, la consommation de *delta*-9-THC était relativement faible, aucun pays ne déclarant une consommation supérieure à 0,3 S-DDD$_{ptpd}$. À partir de 2022, la consommation a augmenté, notamment en Australie, qui a déclaré 0,62 S-DDD$_{ptpd}$ cette année-là, alors que les autres pays ont déclaré moins de 0,3 S-DDD$_{ptpd}$. En 2023, la consommation a fortement augmenté, l'Afrique du Sud ayant déclaré pour la première fois une consommation (5,53 S-DDD$_{ptpd}$), qui plus est la plus élevée de tous les pays déclarants, suivie par l'Australie (2,05 S-DDD$_{ptpd}$), le Portugal (0,17 S-DDD$_{ptpd}$), l'Autriche (0,06 S-DDD$_{ptpd}$), la Suisse (0,05 S-DDD$_{ptpd}$) et le Royaume-Uni (0,05 S-DDD$_{ptpd}$).

Hallucinogènes

Méthylènedioxy-3,4 méthamphétamine

18. La MDMA est un stimulant aux propriétés empathogènes, entactogènes et légèrement hallucinogènes qui est inscrite au Tableau I de la Convention de 1971. Depuis que la MDMA a été placée sous contrôle international au milieu des années 80, son utilisation licite a surtout été limitée à la recherche scientifique et clinique. Ces dernières années, quelques pays ont autorisé à titre exceptionnel l'utilisation de la MDMA pour traiter des troubles mentaux spécifiques liés à des traumatismes, y compris le trouble de stress post-traumatique.

19. Les activités licites liées à la MDMA ont été limitées entre le moment où la substance a été placée sous contrôle international et 2019, date à laquelle la fabrication et la consommation de la substance ont augmenté, probablement en raison de l'intensification de la recherche sur des applications thérapeutiques possibles. La MDMA n'est fabriquée que dans quelques pays, bien que la fabrication totale de 25,54 kg déclarée pour 2023 soit la plus grosse quantité fabriquée au cours des 10 dernières années. Le Royaume-Uni a déclaré en avoir fabriqué 22,34 kg, suivi par le Canada avec 2,68 kg. L'Australie, les États-Unis, les Pays-Bas (Royaume des) et la Suisse ont également signalé de très faibles quantités. Depuis qu'il a augmenté sa fabrication de MDMA en 2020, le Royaume-Uni est également le principal détenteur de stocks de cette substance, avec environ 12 kg déclarés chaque année depuis 2021. Les stocks mondiaux de MDMA s'élevaient à 17,01 kg en 2023 (voir fig. 5).

20. Au total, 22 pays et territoires ont déclaré des importations de MDMA en 2023, mais, comme les années précédentes, il s'agissait de très faibles quantités. Les exportations de MDMA ont également été limitées : le Canada, premier exportateur, a déclaré avoir exporté 0,67 kg en 2023. Dans l'ensemble, le commerce de la MDMA est resté pratiquement inchangé ces 10 dernières années.

21. La consommation totale de MDMA en 2023 s'élevait à 16,67 kg, mais elle était presque entièrement concentrée au Royaume-Uni (15,87 kg)[2]. Le Canada, la Suisse et Israël ont été les autres principaux consommateurs, avec respectivement 0,24 kg, 0,21 kg et 0,18 kg.

Psilocybine et psilocine

22. La psilocybine et la psilocine (psilotsine) sont des substances hallucinogènes inscrites au Tableau I de la Convention de 1971. Elles existent toutes deux à l'état naturel et sont présentes dans de nombreuses espèces de champignons poussant dans toutes les régions du monde. La psilocybine est un précurseur qui se transforme en psilocine dans le corps humain. Comme dans le cas de la MDMA, les activités licites liées à la psilocybine et à la psilocine ont été très limitées depuis leur placement sous contrôle international, mais comme au cours

[2] La consommation de méthylènedioxy-3,4 méthamphétamine (MDMA) ne peut être exprimée qu'en termes de poids brut, car aucune S-DDD n'a été établie pour cette substance.

Figure 5. MDMA : fabrication, stocks et consommation (2014-2023)

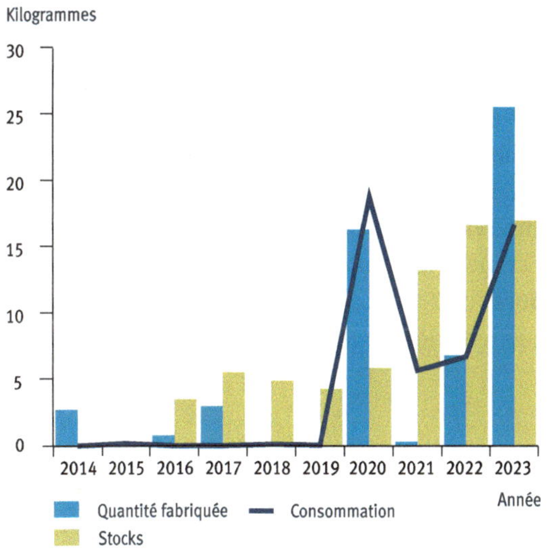

Figure 6. Fabrication de psilocybine et de psilocine (2014-2023)

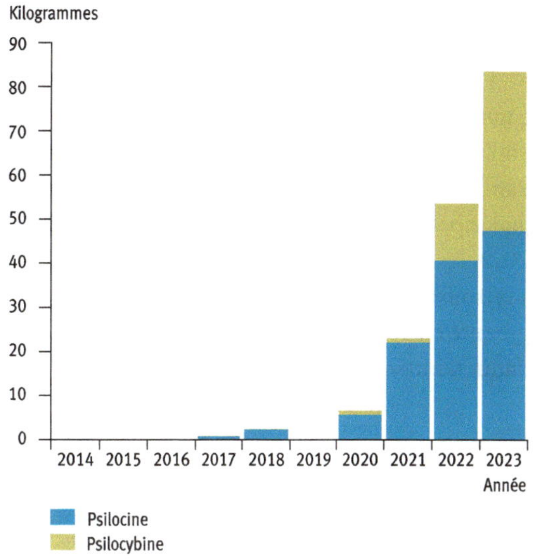

des dernières années de plus en plus de pays ont autorisé la recherche et les essais cliniques les concernant, on a constaté une augmentation des activités licites liées à leur fabrication, à leur commerce et à leur consommation.

23. Avant 2020, la fabrication de psilocybine et de psilocine était très limitée, la production mondiale totale ne dépassant pas quelques dizaines de grammes. En 2020, la fabrication mondiale totale de psilocybine a augmenté pour atteindre environ 1 kg et n'a que légèrement évolué en 2021. En 2022, elle est passée à 13 kg, puis à 36,1 kg en 2023 (voir fig. 6). En 2022 et 2023, le Royaume-Uni a été le principal fabricant de psilocybine, déclarant respectivement 8,9 kg et 30,9 kg. Le Canada, les États-Unis et les Pays-Bas (Royaume des) sont les seuls autres pays à avoir déclaré une fabrication significative en 2022 et 2023.

24. Comme pour la fabrication, le commerce de la psilocybine et de la psilocine est resté très limité jusqu'en 2020. Avant, les quantités échangées déclarées par les pays et territoires dépassaient rarement quelques grammes. En 2020, les importations mondiales totales de psilocybine et de psilocine s'élevaient respectivement à 0,46 kg et 0,04 kg. En ce qui concerne la psilocybine, le chiffre est passé à environ 1 kg en 2021 et a fortement augmenté en 2022, pour atteindre 7,91 kg. En 2023, les importations mondiales de psilocybine sont restées stables à 7,8 kg. En ce qui concerne la psilocine, les importations mondiales totales ont atteint 0,04 kg en 2020 et sont restées pratiquement inchangées depuis. En 2023, les importations mondiales totales de cette substance s'élevaient à 0,06 kg.

25. La consommation de psilocine n'a été signalée par aucun pays ou territoires au cours de la dernière décennie. Historiquement, la consommation de psilocybine a été limitée à quelques dizaines de grammes signalés par quelques pays seulement. En 2022, la consommation mondiale a augmenté de manière significative, atteignant 1,3 kg, principalement en raison de l'augmentation de la consommation au Royaume-Uni (0,64 kg), en Allemagne (0,25 kg) et aux États-Unis (0,25 kg)[3]. La consommation mondiale totale de psilocybine a encore augmenté pour atteindre 3,86 kg en 2023, le Royaume-Uni (3,1 kg) comptant pour la majeure partie, devant les États-Unis (0,46 kg) et l'Australie (0,13 kg). Six autres pays ont déclaré une consommation de cette substance, mais en très petites quantités.

Amphétamines

26. Six amphétamines sont inscrites au Tableau II de la Convention de 1971 : les deux isomères optiques de l'amfétamine (lévamfétamine et dexamfétamine) et leur mélange racémique (amfétamine), ainsi que les deux

[3] La consommation de psilocybine ne peut être exprimée qu'en termes de poids brut, car aucune S-DDD n'a été établie pour cette substance.

Français

isomères optiques de la métamfétamine (lévométhamphétamine et métamfétamine) et leur mélange racémique (racémate de métamfétamine). Certaines de ces substances, en particulier la dexamfétamine, sont généralement utilisées pour traiter les personnes souffrant d'un trouble du déficit de l'attention avec ou sans hyperactivité (TDAH).

27. En 2023, trois amphétamines (amfétamine, dexamfétamine et métamfétamine) étaient présentes en quantité non négligeable sur le marché licite et 42 pays et territoires en ont importé au moins une (voir tableau 4). Parmi ces trois substances, la dexamfétamine est celle qui a été fabriquée en plus grande quantité. La quantité de dexamfétamine fabriquée dans le monde a augmenté cette année-là, principalement en raison de l'augmentation signalée par les États-Unis. La fabrication mondiale d'amfétamine est restée pratiquement inchangée entre 2022 et 2023, les États-Unis en étant le seul fabricant. En ce qui concerne la métamfétamine, les quantités fabriquées ont retrouvé les niveaux de 2021 après avoir été très peu fabriquées en 2022. Le commerce des trois substances a augmenté entre 2022 et 2023, principalement en raison de l'augmentation des importations d'amfétamine et de dexamfétamine signalée par l'Allemagne.

Tableau 4. Amphétamines présentes en quantité non négligeable sur le marché licite (classées en fonction des quantités fabriquées) : fabrication et importations mondiales totales, et nombre de pays et territoires importateurs (2023)

Substance	*S-DDD (en mg)*	*Quantité fabriquée (en kg)*	*Importations (en kg)*	*Nombre de pays et territoires importateurs*
Dexamfétamine	15	47 461,41	5 869,54	42
Amfétamine	15	16 766,23	835,63	31
Métamfétamine	15	596,89	1 200,37	24

Dexamfétamine

28. La fabrication totale de dexamfétamine est passée de 40 tonnes en 2022 à 47,5 tonnes en 2023 (voir fig. 7), les États-Unis ayant déclaré une augmentation de 10 tonnes par rapport à l'année précédente. Comme c'est le cas depuis de nombreuses années, les États-Unis ont été le plus gros fabricant de dexamfétamine en 2023, avec 42,6 tonnes. Ils sont suivis du Danemark (4,8 tonnes) et de la Finlande (84,1 kg). La France, qui a toujours été un important fabricant de dexamfétamine et d'amfétamine, s'est retirée du marché et n'a pas déclaré la fabrication de quelque type d'amphétamine que ce soit depuis 2019.

Figure 7. Dexamfétamine : fabrication, importations et stocks dans le monde (2014–2023)

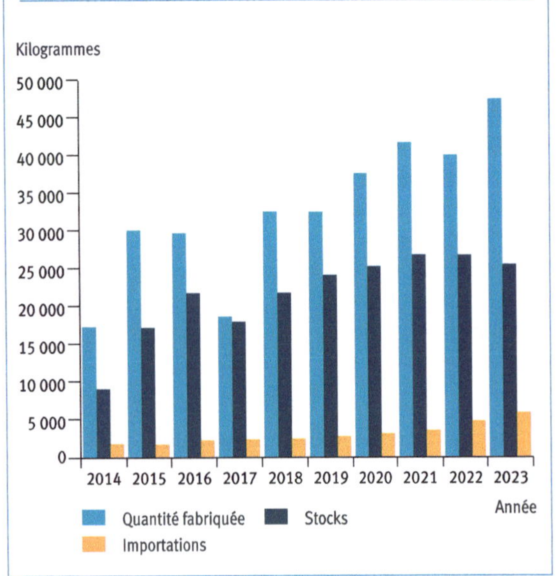

Figure 8. Dexamfétamine : quantités utilisées pour la fabrication de substances non psychotropes (2014-2023)

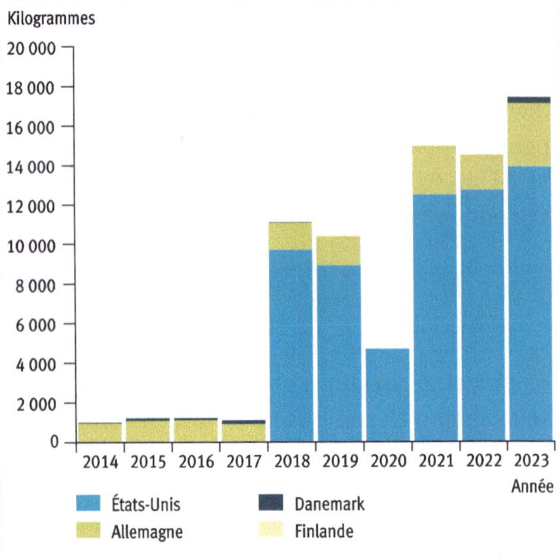

29. Les importations mondiales de dexamfétamine ont augmenté régulièrement au cours des 10 dernières années, passant de 1,79 tonne en 2014 à 5,69 tonnes en 2023, 41 pays et territoires en ayant déclaré des importations en 2023. Le plus grand importateur était l'Allemagne, avec 3,46 tonnes, suivie de l'Australie (601,1 kg), du Canada (505,9 kg), du Royaume des Pays-Bas (265,1 kg) et du Chili (237 kg). Les principaux importateurs de cette substance sont donc restés les mêmes qu'en 2022. Les exportations totales sont passées de 3,66 tonnes en 2022 à 4,41 tonnes en 2023, principalement en raison d'une augmentation des exportations déclarées par le Danemark (premier pays exportateur avec 3,08 tonnes), suivi par la France (449,8 kg), les États-Unis (350,9 kg), l'Allemagne (326,1 kg) et la Croatie (108,4 kg).

30. En 2023, 27 pays ont déclaré une consommation de dexamfétamine. La consommation globale a augmenté par rapport à l'année précédente dans la plupart de ces pays. L'Australie a fourni des données sur la consommation de la substance pour la première fois en 2023. Les principaux consommateurs de dexamfétamine en 2023 étaient les États-Unis (11,50 S-DDD$_{ptpd}$), l'Australie (4,25 S-DDD$_{ptpd}$), Israël (2,57 S-DDD$_{ptpd}$) et le Canada (2,04 S-DDD$_{ptpd}$). Tous les autres pays ayant communiqué des données ont déclaré une consommation inférieure à 2 S-DDD$_{ptpd}$. Les 10 pays et territoires ayant déclaré les taux de consommation de dexamfétamine les plus élevés en 2023 sont répertoriés dans le tableau 5.

Tableau 5. Dexamfétamine : taux de consommation des 10 pays ayant déclaré les niveaux de consommation les plus élevés en 2023, et comparaison avec 2021 et 2022

	S-DDD par millier d'habitants et par jour		
Pays	*2021*	*2022*	*2023*
États-Unis	8,57	8,05	11,50
Australie	–	–	4,25
Israël	1,52	2,07	2,57
Canada	1,60	1,90	2,04
Chili	0,53	0,78	1,58
Islande	0,91	0,94	1,27
Pays-Bas (Royaume des)	1,10	1,26	1,26
Norvège	–	1,00	1,14
Suède	0,92	0,89	0,92
Nouvelle-Zélande	0,58	0,07	0,58

31. Aux États-Unis, la dexamfétamine est aussi utilisée dans la synthèse de la lisdexamfétamine (l-lysine-d-amfétamine), un précurseur de la dexamfétamine qui n'est pas placé sous contrôle international et qui est utilisé dans le traitement du TDAH. Les États-Unis ont commencé à déclarer l'utilisation de dexamfétamine pour la fabrication de substances non psychotropes en 2018, et la quantité utilisée n'a cessé d'augmenter depuis. En 2023, 17,4 tonnes de dexamfétamine ont été utilisées pour la fabrication de substances non psychotropes, principalement par les États-Unis (13,9 tonnes). Selon les informations fournies à l'OICS, cette quantité a été entièrement utilisée pour la fabrication de lisdexamfétamine. L'Allemagne et le Danemark ont également signalé l'utilisation de dexamfétamine pour la fabrication de substances non psychotropes en 2023, avec respectivement 3,2 tonnes et 302 kg (voir fig. 8).

ENCADRÉ 2. PRÉCURSEUR DE LA DEXAMFÉTAMINE : LISDEXAMFÉTAMINE

Un précurseur est un composé inactif qui devient actif une fois métabolisé dans l'organisme, libérant son composant actif pour exercer ses effets. C'est le cas de la lisdexamfétamine (l-lysine-d-amfétamine), un précurseur de la dexamfétamine, qui est un stimulant du système nerveux central inscrit au Tableau II de la Convention sur les substances psychotropes de 1971.

La lisdexamfétamine a fait l'objet d'un examen préalable par le Comité d'experts de la pharmacodépendance de l'Organisation mondiale de la Santé à sa trente-sixième réunion, en juin 2014. Dans son rapport, le Comité a déclaré que la sécurité et l'efficacité de la lisdexamfétamine dans le traitement du trouble du déficit de l'attention avec ou sans hyperactivité (TDAH) avaient été établies.

ENCADRÉ 2. PRÉCURSEUR DE LA DEXAMFÉTAMINE : LISDEXAMFÉTAMINE *(suite)*

Dans le même temps, il a conclu que le fait que la lisdexamfétamine soit un précurseur de la dexamfétamine impliquait la nécessité d'une surveillance clinique et de précautions similaires pour le suivi et la programmation de ce stimulant du système nerveux central. La substance n'a jamais atteint la deuxième étape de la procédure d'examen (examen critique).

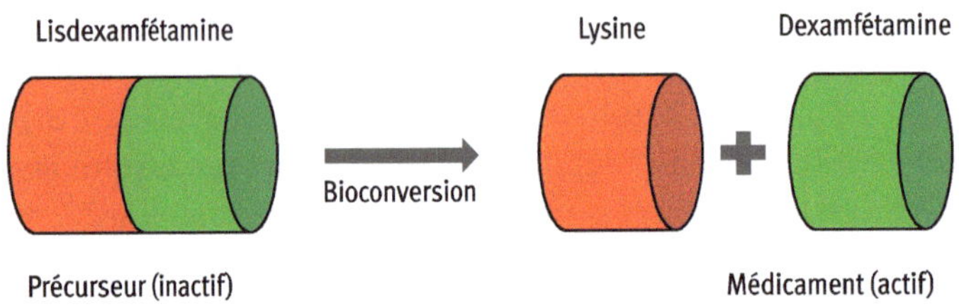

Principalement utilisée dans le traitement du TDAH, la lisdexamfétamine a gagné en importance depuis sa commercialisation en 2007 et a été mise sur le marché sous différents noms de marque, tels que Vyvanse. Lorsqu'elle est administrée par voie orale et métabolisée dans le corps humain, la substance est décomposée en lysine, un acide aminé, et en dexamfétamine. La lisdexamfétamine présente un potentiel d'usage abusif plus faible que la dexamfétamine et ne fait actuellement pas l'objet d'un contrôle international. Par conséquent, les autorités compétentes ne sont pas tenues de la surveiller et de communiquer des données statistiques à l'Organe international de contrôle des stupéfiants comme elles le font pour les substances psychotropes placées sous contrôle international. Toutefois, certains pays ont placé cette substance sous contrôle national.

Des données récentes montrent que la fabrication mondiale de lisdexamfétamine suit une tendance à la hausse, en particulier aux États-Unis, qui comptaient pour 90 % de la fabrication mondiale de dexamfétamine en 2023 et ont déclaré que 33 % de la substance avait été utilisée pour fabriquer de la lisdexamfétamine. Certains pays européens, dont l'Allemagne et le Danemark, ont également constaté une augmentation du commerce de la dexamfétamine. L'Allemagne a signalé une utilisation croissante de la substance pour la fabrication de substances psychotropes non contrôlées. L'OICS a également observé un intérêt croissant pour la lisdexamfétamine de la part de la Bolivie (État plurinational de), de la Croatie et du Panama.

La lisdexamfétamine n'étant actuellement pas soumise à un contrôle international, les données dont dispose l'OICS sont fournies par les pays sur la base du volontariat et ne reflètent donc pas la situation mondiale. Néanmoins, sur la base des données fournies et des demandes reçues par différents pays concernant la lisdexamfétamine, il semble que la substance soit de plus en plus présente sur le marché international licite. Avec le temps, la consommation de dexamfétamine à des fins médicales pourrait être remplacée par celle de lisdexamfétamine.

L'OICS remercie les pays qui ont volontairement communiqué des informations sur la lisdexamfétamine et encourage tous les pays et territoires à communiquer à l'avenir des informations sur les exportations et les importations de cette substance.

Amfétamine

32. La fabrication totale d'amfétamine a légèrement augmenté, passant de 16,1 tonnes en 2022 à 16,8 tonnes en 2023 (voir fig. 9). Comme les années précédentes, les États-Unis ont été le principal fabricant de la substance, à l'exception de quelques grammes fabriqués par plusieurs autres pays. Les stocks mondiaux d'amfétamine ont baissé, passant de 22,5 tonnes en 2022 à 19,6 tonnes en 2023. La plus grosse partie de ces stocks se trouvaient aux États-Unis (19,2 tonnes). Le Canada a été l'autre grand détenteur de stocks et a déclaré 257,9 kg. La France, qui détenait depuis toujours d'importants stocks d'amfétamine, a déclaré un total de 12,4 kg pour 2023.

33. Le commerce de l'amfétamine est relativement limité par rapport à celui d'autres substances psychotropes. Depuis 2018, les importations d'amfétamine n'ont pas dépassé 1 tonne. Pour 2023, les importations mondiales

Figure 9. Amfétamine : fabrication, importations et stocks dans le monde (2014–2023)

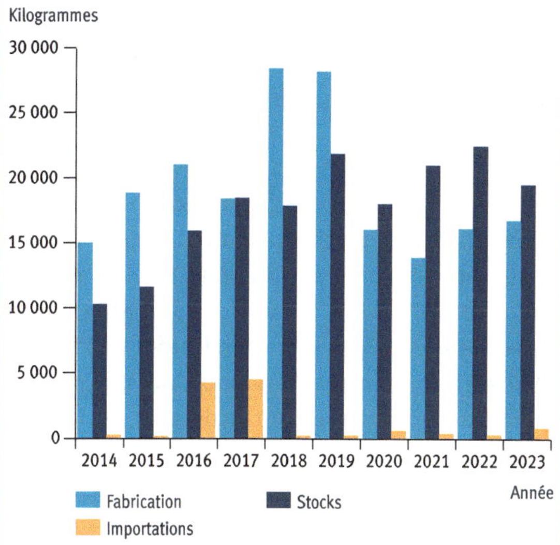

s'élevaient à 835,6 kg, l'Allemagne (560,7 kg) et le Canada (239,3 kg) comptant pour la quasi-totalité. Vingt-neuf autres pays ont signalé des importations de la substance, mais seulement quelques kilogrammes ou moins. En tant que premier fabricant d'amfétamine, les États-Unis en ont également été le principal exportateur, déclarant 1,3 tonne en 2023, contre 961,8 kg en 2022. Dix autres pays ont signalé des exportations, mais seulement quelques kilogrammes ou moins.

34. En 2023, 15 pays et territoires au total ont déclaré une consommation d'amfétamine. La consommation globale a légèrement augmenté, principalement en raison d'une hausse aux États-Unis, mais de nombreux pays et territoires ont fait état d'une consommation inférieure à celle de l'année précédente. Les cinq pays et territoires en ayant consommé les plus grosses quantités ont été les États-Unis (10,51 S-DDD_{ptpd}), le Canada (0,98 S-DDD_{ptpd}), les Îles Turques et Caïques (0,27 S-DDD_{ptpd}), la Norvège (0,10 S-DDD_{ptpd}) et la Suède (0,09 S-DDD_{ptpd}).

Français

Métamfétamine

35. La fabrication mondiale de métamfétamine est passée de quelques grammes en 2022 à 596,8 kg en 2023. La Hongrie a déclaré avoir fabriqué de la métamfétamine pour la première fois depuis 2020 et assuré la quasi-totalité de la fabrication de cette substance en 2023. Deux autres pays en ont signalé la fabrication de quelques grammes. Les stocks mondiaux de métamfétamine ont diminué, passant de 2,1 tonnes en 2022 à 243,5 kg en 2023, la France n'ayant pas déclaré de stocks. La Hongrie détenait la quasi-totalité des stocks mondiaux.

36. Pendant plusieurs années, le commerce de la métamfétamine était minime, avec seulement quelques grammes importés ou exportés chaque année. En 2023, cependant, les importations et les exportations mondiales ont augmenté de 1,2 tonne chacune, en raison de l'exportation de cette quantité de la France vers les États-Unis en cours d'année. Les autres échanges de métamfétamine sont restés limités, quelques autres pays ayant déclaré des exportations et des importations de quelques grammes seulement.

37. La consommation de métamfétamine n'est signalée que par quelques pays, et en très faibles quantités. Le seul pays à déclarer une consommation significative en 2023 a été la Macédoine du Nord (0,01 S-DDD_{ptpd}). La Nouvelle-Zélande, qui avait déclaré une consommation les années précédentes, n'en a déclaré aucune en 2023.

Méthylphénidate

38. Comme les amphétamines, le méthylphénidate est un stimulant inscrit au Tableau II de la Convention de 1971 et il est également utilisé pour le traitement du TDAH. Parmi les stimulants inscrits au Tableau II, c'est celui qui est le plus largement fabriqué et commercialisé, 120 pays et territoires en ayant déclaré des importations en 2023 (voir tableau 6).

Tableau 6. Méthylphénidate : fabrication et importations mondiales totales, et nombre de pays et territoires importateurs (2022 et 2023)

Année	*S-DDD (en mg)*	*Quantité fabriquée (en kg)*	*Importations (en kg)*	*Nombre de pays et territoires importateurs*
2022	30	64 539,54	52 406,76	117
2023	30	82 645,73	59 952,31	120

Figure 10. Méthylphénidate: fabrication, importations et stocks dans le monde, (2014–2023)

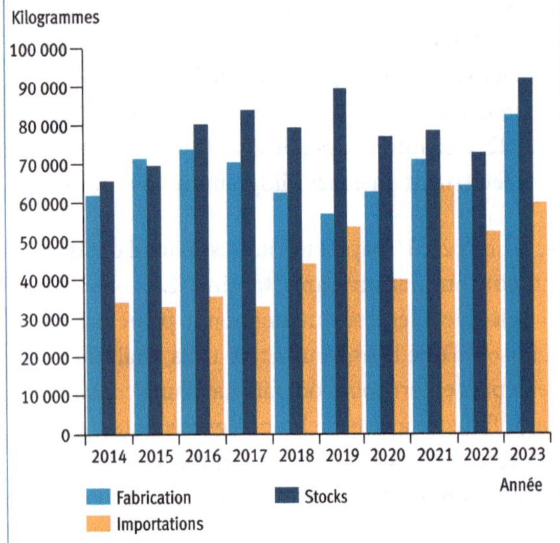

39. La fabrication mondiale de méthylphénidate a amorcé une croissance en 2012 et atteint 74 tonnes en 2016, le plus haut niveau observé depuis les années 90. En 2017, elle a commencé à fléchir, pour s'établir à 57,2 tonnes en 2019. La fabrication totale s'est ensuite reprise pour atteindre 82,6 tonnes en 2023, niveau le plus élevé depuis les premières données reçues par l'OICS (voir fig. 10).

40. L'augmentation de la fabrication totale de méthylphénidate a principalement résulté des augmentations signalées par les États-Unis, l'Inde et la Suisse. En 2023, les États-Unis (58,4 tonnes) ont de nouveau été le premier fabricant. L'Inde (11,2 tonnes), la Suisse (6,6 tonnes), le Royaume-Uni (4,7 tonnes) et l'Espagne (1,1 tonne) en ont également fabriqué des quantités importantes.

41. Les stocks mondiaux de méthylphénidate ont augmenté de près de 20 tonnes, passant de 72,9 tonnes en 2022 à 92 tonnes en 2023. Cette augmentation peut être attribuée principalement au Royaume-Uni, dont les stocks sont passés de 2,9 tonnes à 17 tonnes, et à l'Allemagne, dont les stocks sont passés de 6,8 tonnes à 8,9 tonnes. En 2023, et comme les années précédentes, les États-Unis (44,5 tonnes) ont compté pour près de la moitié des stocks mondiaux. Le Royaume-Uni (17 tonnes), l'Allemagne (8,9 tonnes), la Suisse (7,6 tonnes) et le Canada (4 tonnes) étaient les autres principaux détenteurs de stocks de méthylphénidate.

42. Le commerce international de méthylphénidate est resté très actif en 2023, 120 pays et territoires ayant déclaré des importations de cette substance et une quantité croissante de méthylphénidate fabriqué aux États-Unis ayant été exportée vers d'autres pays.

43. Le volume des importations de méthylphénidate déclaré par les pays et territoires a augmenté, passant de 52,4 tonnes en 2022 à 60 tonnes en 2023. Cette augmentation peut être attribuée en grande partie à des hausses modestes des importations par les principaux importateurs. Les cinq principaux importateurs de méthylphénidate en 2023 étaient l'Allemagne (10,5 tonnes), le Canada (6,3 tonnes), la Suisse (5,8 tonnes), l'Espagne (5,5 tonnes) et la Belgique (3,5 tonnes). Treize autres pays en ont déclaré des importations de plus d'une tonne. Parmi les autres pays et territoires en ayant déclaré des importations en 2023, 48 en ont importé plus de 10 kg.

44. Le volume total des importations de méthylphénidate déclaré par les pays et territoires a augmenté, passant de 49,8 tonnes en 2022 à 60,9 tonnes en 2023. Les États-Unis étaient les principaux exportateurs, avec 17,4 tonnes, contre 15,8 tonnes en 2022. Les autres principaux exportateurs étaient la Suisse (9,1 tonnes), l'Inde (8,7 tonnes), le Royaume-Uni (6,1 tonnes), l'Allemagne (5,9 tonnes) et l'Espagne (5,1 tonnes).

45. L'usage du méthylphénidate à des fins médicales a considérablement augmenté dans les années 90. Cette substance est utilisée pour le traitement du TDAH, principalement chez les enfants. Elle est également prescrite pour le traitement de la narcolepsie. La hausse de sa fabrication et de son utilisation s'explique principalement par la situation aux États-Unis, où cette substance est souvent prescrite dans le traitement du TDAH et fait l'objet de campagnes publicitaires intenses, qui s'adressent directement aux consommateurs et consommatrices potentiels.

46. Le nombre de pays et territoires ayant déclaré une consommation de méthylphénidate a augmenté, passant de 66 en 2022 à 80 en 2023. La différence entre les taux de consommation les plus élevés et les plus faibles restait considérable, principalement en raison d'une quantité importante déclarée par l'Islande, qui a toujours affiché des niveaux élevés de consommation de méthylphénidate depuis de nombreuses années.

47. Comparativement aux chiffres communiqués pour 2022, la consommation de cette substance a augmenté en Islande, où elle est passée de 29,47 S-DDD$_{ptpd}$ à 34,5 S-DDD$_{ptpd}$; le pays a déclaré la plus forte consommation mondiale en 2023, comme c'est le cas depuis de nombreuses années. La consommation de cette substance a légèrement augmenté dans presque tous les pays qui ont fourni des données (voir tableau 7).

Tableau 7. Méthylphénidate : consommation des 10 pays ayant déclaré les niveaux de consommation les plus élevés en 2023, et comparaison avec 2021 et 2022

	S-DDD par millier d'habitants et par jour		
Pays	*2021*	*2022*	*2023*
Islande	53,33	29,47	34,50
Danemark	9,39	10,63	12,88
Canada	10,01	11,14	12,15
Nouvelle-Zélande	7,70	5,35	9,87
Suède	8,57	9,01	9,61
Norvège	–	8,38	9,14
Pays-Bas (Royaume des)	7,74	8,33	9,11
Israël	10,05	7,73	8,36
États-Unis	7,34	6,90	7,14
Australie	–	–	6,38

Phentermine

48. Des stimulants inscrits au Tableau II de la Convention de 1971, un seul (la phentermine) était présent en quantité non négligeable sur le marché licite en 2023. La phentermine est restée le stimulant non amphétaminique le plus fabriqué et elle est utilisée médicalement comme coupe-faim dans la prise en charge ponctuelle de l'obésité.

49. La quantité qui en a été fabriquée dans le monde a continué de diminuer en 2023, principalement en raison des baisses déclarées par l'Allemagne. Le volume des importations a augmenté en 2023 en raison d'une hausse significative des importations par les États-Unis. Au total, 43 pays et territoires ont déclaré des importations de phentermine en 2023 (voir tableau 8). Les tendances en matière de consommation sont restées largement inchangées, la Nouvelle-Zélande et le Chili étant les plus gros consommateurs par habitant en 2023.

Tableau 8. Phentermine : fabrication et importations mondiales totales, 2023

Substance	*S-DDD (en mg)*	*Quantité fabriquée (en kg)*	*Importations (en kg)*	*Nombre de pays et territoires importateurs*
Phentermine	15	26 551,94	24 014,82	43

50. La fabrication mondiale de phentermine a reculé pour la deuxième année consécutive, passant de 29,1 tonnes en 2022 à 26,6 tonnes en 2023, en raison d'une réduction de 9 tonnes en glissement annuel signalée par les États-Unis, tandis que l'Allemagne a fait état d'une augmentation de 7 tonnes. L'Allemagne était le premier fabricant de phentermine en 2023, avec 19,3 tonnes, suivie des États-Unis (3,7 tonnes), de l'Italie (2,38 tonnes) et de l'Inde (675,1 kg). Les stocks mondiaux de phentermine ont également diminué pour la deuxième année consécutive, passant de 27,5 tonnes en 2022 à 23,3 tonnes en 2023. La plus grosse part des stocks était détenue par les États-Unis (13,9 tonnes), suivis par l'Allemagne (4,6 tonnes) et l'Italie (1 tonne). Vingt et un autres pays ont déclaré en détenir, en petites quantités.

51. Les importations mondiales de phentermine ont augmenté en 2023, 43 pays et territoires ayant déclaré un total de 24 tonnes importées, contre 19,4 tonnes en 2022. Comme en 2022, les États-Unis en sont restés le premier importateur (9,2 tonnes), suivis du Mexique (5 tonnes), du Chili (2,7 tonnes) et de la République de Corée (1,7 tonnes). Les exportations mondiales de phentermine ont augmenté pour s'établir à 24,6 tonnes en 2023, l'Allemagne en restant le principal exportateur (17 tonnes). Les autres gros exportateurs étaient l'Italie (2,8 tonnes), l'Australie (962,4 kg), l'Inde (946,5 kg), la Suisse (888,6 kg) et les États-Unis (887,5 kg).

52. Vingt-cinq pays et territoires ont communiqué des données sur la consommation de phentermine en 2023, la Nouvelle-Zélande (14,35 $S\text{-}DDD_{ptpd}$), le Chili (9,18 $S\text{-}DDD_{ptpd}$), les États-Unis (8,56 $S\text{-}DDD_{ptpd}$), le Mexique (8,31 $S\text{-}DDD_{ptpd}$) et la République de Corée (7,95 $S\text{-}DDD_{ptpd}$) affichant les cinq taux de consommation les plus élevés, tout comme l'année précédente. Bien que les pays où la consommation de phentermine est la plus élevée soient les mêmes qu'en 2022, la consommation globale a diminué dans tous les pays et territoires en 2023.

Benzodiazépines

53. Les benzodiazépines sont une classe de substances inscrites au Tableau IV de la Convention de 1971, utilisées pour le traitement d'un ensemble d'affections. Certaines des benzodiazépines le plus couramment prescrites sont utilisées pour traiter l'anxiété, les troubles paniques, la dépression et l'insomnie, et certaines sont également utilisées pour l'anesthésie générale, la sédation avant une intervention chirurgicale, le sevrage alcoolique et l'agitation associée à l'usage de drogues. Les benzodiazépines font l'objet d'un commerce mondial depuis de nombreuses décennies. Au cours de la période 2014-2023, presque tous les pays et territoires ont déclaré à l'OICS le commerce d'au moins une benzodiazépine en quantité supérieure à 1 kg.

54. Les premières benzodiazépines ont été placées sous contrôle international au début des années 80. Au fil du temps, les mesures de contrôle ont été étendues à d'autres substances et, à l'heure actuelle, 41 benzodiazépines font l'objet d'un contrôle international, dont quatre en tant que nouvelles substances psychoactives.

55. Sur les 41 benzodiazépines sous contrôle international, 16 étaient présentes en quantité non négligeable sur le marché licite en 2023 (voir tableau 9). Comme les années précédentes, le diazépam, le midazolam, le clonazépam, l'alprazolam et le lorazépam ont été les benzodiazépines ayant fait le plus l'objet d'un commerce en 2023, chacune ayant été importée par au moins 126 pays et territoires. Par rapport à 2022, le nombre de pays et territoires qui ont déclaré en importer n'a que très peu changé.

Tableau 9. Benzodiazépines présentes en quantité non négligeable sur le marché licite : quantités totales fabriquées dans le monde et nombre de pays et territoires importateurs (classés en fonction des quantités fabriquées en S-DDD) (2023)

Substance	*S-DDD (en mg)*	*Quantité fabriquée (en kg)*	*Quantité fabriquée (en millions de S-DDD)*	*Nombre de pays et territoires importateurs*
Alprazolam	1	15 550,22	15 550,22	139
Diazépam	10	58 226,30	5 822,63	164
Clonazépam	4	17 938,95	4 484,74	142
Lorazépam	2,5	10 198,60	4 079,44	126
Bromazépam	10	8 959,04	895,90	113
Chlordiazépoxide	30	22 826,23	760,87	83
Midazolam	15	9 157,37	610,49	159
Nitrazépam	5	2 860,76	572,15	54
Flunitrazépam	1	543,73	543,73	31
Clobazam	20	8 734,77	436,74	95
Oxazépam	50	18 799,45	375,99	53
Témazépam	20	6 853,11	342,66	32
Triazolam	0,25	57,70	230,79	39
Prazépam	30	3 900,33	130,01	27
Flurazépam	30	2 757,74	91,92	21
Clorazépate	20	1 486,93	74,35	44

56. En 2023, la quantité totale fabriquée des benzodiazépines ayant une présence importante sur le marché illicite a atteint environ 189 tonnes, ce qui représente une augmentation par rapport à 2022. Si la fabrication a été déclarée dans plusieurs régions du monde, 96 % du total a été concentré dans quatre pays, à savoir l'Italie (41 %), l'Inde (37 %), la Chine (9 %) et le Brésil (9 %). Malgré une légère baisse de la production, l'Italie est restée le premier producteur. En Inde, la fabrication a augmenté de 31 % par rapport à 2022 et atteint un niveau record, tandis que la Chine a presque doublé sa fabrication entre 2022 et 2023. En termes de poids brut, huit benzodiazépines — diazépam, chlordiazépoxide, oxazépam, clonazépam, alprazolam, lorazépam, midazolam et bromazépam — ont représenté 86 % de la fabrication totale en 2023 (voir fig. 11).

Figure 11. Benzodiazépines présentes en quantité non négligeable sur le marché licite : répartition de la fabrication mondiale, par substance, sur la base du poids brut (2023)

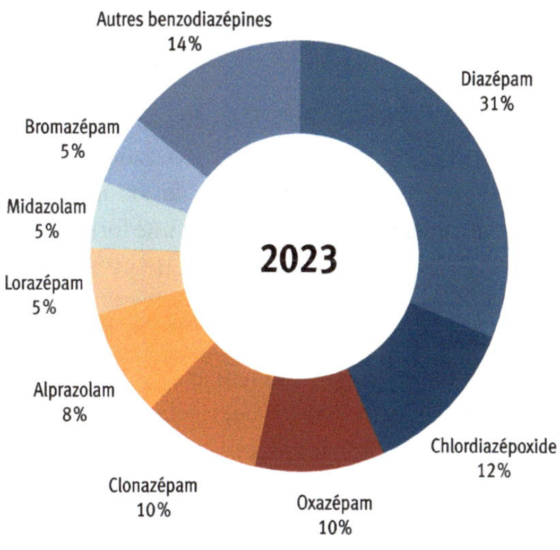

Figure 12. Diazépam : nombre de pays et territoires ayant déclaré la consommation de cette substance, par région (2019-2023)

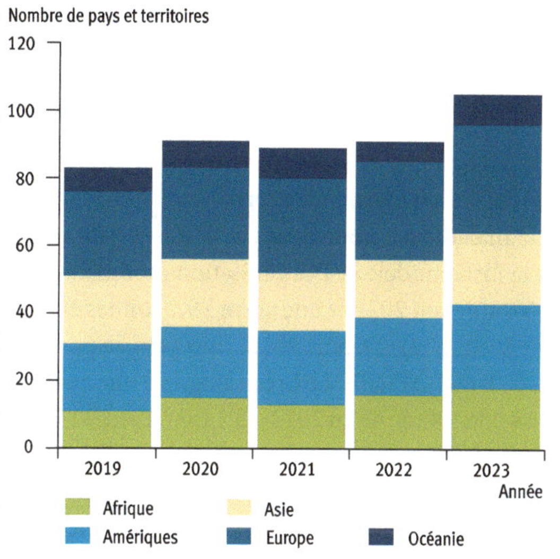

Diazépam

57. Le diazépam a été la benzodiazépine la plus fabriquée en 2023, en poids brut (58,2 tonnes), puisqu'il a représenté 31 % de la quantité totale fabriquée des benzodiazépines présentes en quantité non négligeable sur le marché licite. La quantité de diazépam fabriquée au niveau mondial a connu de fortes fluctuations ces dernières années. La fabrication de cette substance en Italie a atteint un record avec 29,2 tonnes en 2021, avant de fortement diminuer, tombant à 17,9 tonnes en 2023. En revanche, l'Inde a considérablement augmenté sa fabrication, passant de 12,7 tonnes en 2022 à 20,9 tonnes en 2023. En Chine, la fabrication a été instable, tombant à 1,3 tonne en 2020 et remontant à 11,4 tonnes en 2023. Après un creux de 0,4 tonne en 2022, la fabrication au Brésil a rebondi pour atteindre 7,8 tonnes en 2023. Au niveau mondial, plus de 99 % de la fabrication de diazépam en 2023 a été déclarée par quatre pays : Inde, Italie, Chine et Brésil. Le total des stocks détenus par l'ensemble des pays et territoires fabriquant du diazépam a légèrement diminué entre 2022 et 2023, passant de 42,9 tonnes à 40,3 tonnes. Les pays détenant les plus gros stocks de cette substance en 2023 étaient la Chine (10,4 tonnes), l'Italie (8,3 tonnes), le Brésil (6,2 tonnes) et le Danemark (3,7 tonnes).

58. Le diazépam a également été la substance psychotrope placée sous contrôle international la plus largement échangée en 2023, 164 pays et territoires en ayant déclaré des importations. Les importations mondiales de diazépam avaient augmenté régulièrement, passant de 32,5 tonnes en 2017 à un pic de 66,4 tonnes en 2021. Toutefois, les importations sont ensuite reparties à la baisse, passant à 44,4 tonnes en 2022 et à 37,2 tonnes en 2023. Le nombre de pays et territoires importateurs de diazépam a atteint un nombre record en 2018 (176), avant de fluctuer au cours des années suivantes. Comme indiqué ci-dessus, 164 pays et territoires ont déclaré des importations de la substance en 2023, soit une hausse par rapport à 2022 (160). En 2023, des importations de plus d'une tonne ont été signalées par le Ghana, l'Espagne, les États-Unis, la République démocratique du Congo, la Tchéquie, l'Allemagne, la France, le Bangladesh, le Japon et la Serbie (par ordre décroissant de quantité importée), qui représentaient ensemble environ 60 % du total des importations mondiales. En 2023, les principaux pays exportateurs étaient l'Italie (16,3 tonnes), l'Inde (10,2 tonnes), le Danemark (2,7 tonnes), la Tchéquie (2,2 tonnes), l'Allemagne (1,8 tonne), la Chine (1,7 tonne), la Suisse (1,1 tonne) et l'Espagne (0,7 tonne). Ensemble, ces pays représentaient 93 % des exportations mondiales de cette substance.

59. Parmi les pays et territoires qui ont fourni des données, le nombre de ceux qui ont déclaré des données de consommation pour le diazépam a considérablement augmenté, passant de 91 en 2022 à 105 en 2023 (voir fig. 12). Cabo Verde a déclaré le niveau de consommation de diazépam le plus élevé en 2023, avec 20,90 $S\text{-}DDD_{ptpd}$, ce qui représente une augmentation significative par rapport aux 5,74 $S\text{-}DDD_{ptpd}$ de 2022. Les autres pays à en

avoir déclaré une consommation supérieure à 10 S-DDD$_{ptpd}$ en 2023 ont été le Monténégro (14,37 S-DDD$_{ptpd}$), le Portugal (13,88 S-DDD$_{ptpd}$) et l'Espagne (13,68 S-DDD$_{ptpd}$). Le Brésil a également connu une forte augmentation de sa consommation, celle-ci s'établissant à 12,03 S-DDD$_{ptpd}$ en 2023, contre 1,41 S-DDD$_{ptpd}$ en 2022. La Bosnie-Herzégovine a déclaré un niveau de consommation de 10,71 S-DDD$_{ptpd}$ en 2023, et le Guyana 9,30 S-DDD$_{ptpd}$.

Midazolam

60. La quantité de midazolam fabriquée a atteint un niveau record de 25 tonnes en 2021, cette substance ayant fait l'objet d'une demande accrue en raison de son utilisation comme sédatif pour les patientes et patients atteints de la maladie à coronavirus (COVID-19) admis dans les unités de soins intensifs, ainsi que de son inscription sur la Liste modèle de l'Organisation mondiale de la Santé des médicaments essentiels. Malgré une forte baisse à 13,5 tonnes en 2022 et une autre à 9,2 tonnes en 2023, la quantité fabriquée est restée bien supérieure à ce qu'elle était avant 2021. Depuis 2016, cinq pays se partagent plus de 98 % des quantités fabriquées : le Brésil, la Chine, l'Inde, Israël et l'Italie. Le Brésil a signalé une augmentation significative de sa fabrication de phénobarbital, qui est passée de 1,4 tonne en 2022 à 3,1 tonnes en 2023. En Inde, la fabrication a poursuivi sa tendance à la baisse, passant de 4,4 tonnes en 2022 à 2,9 tonnes en 2023. L'Italie a également enregistré une baisse, fabriquant 2,3 tonnes en 2023, contre 4,4 tonnes en 2022. Israël, fabricant de grosses quantités les années précédentes, n'a rien déclaré en 2023. La Chine a fabriqué 0,8 tonne, contre 0,7 tonne en 2022. Au niveau mondial, les stocks détenus par les fabricants ont diminué en 2023, pour s'établir à 8,4 tonnes, contre 14,4 tonnes en 2022. Les stocks les plus importants étaient détenus par le Brésil (1,8 tonne), l'Italie (1,1 tonne), la France (1,0 tonne), l'Inde (0,9 tonne) et les États-Unis (0,9 tonne). La baisse des stocks mondiaux de midazolam des fabricants, de 14,4 tonnes en 2022 à 8,4 tonnes en 2023, s'explique principalement par des diminutions importantes des stocks au Brésil (de 4,5 tonnes à 1,8 tonne) et en Inde (de 1,4 tonne à 0,9 tonne), entre autres pays.

61. De 2014 à 2023, le volume global des importations de midazolam déclarées dans le monde s'est établi en moyenne à 10,7 tonnes par an. Si le nombre de pays et territoires ayant déclaré des importations est resté relativement stable, le volume des importations a fortement augmenté pour atteindre 18,2 tonnes en 2021, soit son plus haut niveau en 10 ans, en raison une nouvelle fois de la demande liée à la pandémie de COVID-19. En 2022, les importations ont diminué pour s'établir à 12,6 tonnes, suivies d'une nouvelle baisse à 8,6 tonnes déclarées par un total de 159 pays et territoires en 2023. En 2023, le plus gros importateur de midazolam était l'Allemagne (2,9 tonnes) ; les autres pays et territoires ont déclaré des quantités d'importation nettement inférieures. La baisse globale des importations était principalement due à des réductions substantielles de la part des principaux importateurs des années précédentes, tels que le Brésil, qui n'a importé que 0,2 tonne contre 2,5 tonnes en 2022, et la Türkiye, qui a enregistré une baisse drastique de 1,2 tonne en 2022 à seulement 80 kg en 2023. De même, les exportations mondiales de cette substance ont chuté, passant de 20,9 tonnes en 2021 à 12,6 tonnes en 2022 et 9,1 tonnes en 2023. Les principaux exportateurs étaient l'Italie (3,5 tonnes), l'Allemagne (2 tonnes) et l'Inde (1,2 tonne), tandis que d'autres gros exportateurs ont enregistré des baisses nettes. Par exemple, les exportations d'Israël sont passées de 1,9 tonne en 2022 à seulement 471 kg en 2023. De même, les exportations de l'Inde sont passées de 2,8 tonnes en 2022 à 1,2 tonne.

62. Les données de consommation du midazolam pour 2023 ont été fournies par 100 pays et territoires. La Grèce (4,01 S-DDD$_{ptpd}$), Saint-Martin (3,97 S-DDD$_{ptpd}$), le Brésil (3,18 S-DDD$_{ptpd}$) et l'Uruguay (2,30 S-DDD$_{ptpd}$) ont déclaré les taux de consommation de midazolam les plus élevés. Toutefois, de nombreux pays et territoires ont enregistré une baisse significative de la consommation par rapport aux années précédentes. La Grèce, bien qu'en tête de liste, a enregistré une baisse de 7,08 S-DDD$_{ptpd}$ en 2022. De même, la consommation déclarée par la Türkiye, qui avait bondi à 2,34 S-DDD$_{ptpd}$ en 2022, n'était plus que de 0,03 S-DDD$_{ptpd}$ en 2023. Israël a également connu une baisse, sa consommation passant de 1,41 S-DDD$_{ptpd}$ en 2022 à 0,29 S-DDD$_{ptpd}$ en 2023.

Clonazépam

63. Le clonazépam, seule benzodiazépine antiépileptique placée sous contrôle international, est également utilisé pour le traitement des troubles paniques et de l'anxiété. En 2023, la fabrication mondiale de clonazépam a atteint un niveau record. Après une hausse à 17,2 tonnes en 2021, suivie d'une baisse à 10,7 tonnes en 2022, la fabrication totale a bondi à 17,9 tonnes en 2023. L'Inde est le plus gros fabricant, avec 11,4 tonnes en 2023, soit plus du double des 5,2 tonnes déclarées en 2022. Le Brésil suit avec 3,6 tonnes, contre 2,1 tonnes en 2022. L'Italie

(1,6 tonne) et la Chine (1,04 tonne) figurent parmi les autres fabricants importants. La Suisse, qui avait fabriqué d'importantes quantités de clonazépam les années précédentes, n'a déclaré que 3,7 kg en 2022 et rien en 2023. Les stocks de clonazépam ont légèrement diminué, passant de 6,6 tonnes en 2022 à 6,4 tonnes en 2023. En Suisse, les stocks sont passés de 1 tonne en 2022 à 472 kg en 2023. Le Mexique, qui détenait 1 tonne en 2022, n'a rien déclaré en 2023. Dans le même temps, le Brésil a vu ses stocks passer de 1,7 tonne à 2,3 tonnes, ce qui en fait le principal détenteur de stocks de clonazépam en 2023. En Italie, les stocks ont également diminué, de 900 kg en 2022 à 597 kg en 2023.

64. Sur le plan mondial, les importations de clonazépam ont augmenté régulièrement jusqu'en 2022, année où un record de 15,1 tonnes a été atteint. En 2023, cependant, les importations sont tombées à 10,7 tonnes, en grande partie en raison de la réduction significative des importations de l'Allemagne (1,2 tonne, contre 6,8 tonnes en 2022) et de la Suisse (870 kg, contre 1,2 tonne en 2022). En revanche, les États-Unis (1,2 tonne) et le Brésil (960 kg) ont déclaré des niveaux d'importation plus élevés que les années précédentes. L'Espagne n'a pas signalé de changement significatif, avec des importations de 1,1 tonne en 2023, contre 1,2 tonne en 2022.

65. En 2023, 89 pays et territoires ont déclaré des données de consommation pour le clonazépam, alors qu'ils n'étaient que 78 en 2022. Avec 12,79 S-DDD$_{ptpd}$, le Brésil a déclaré la consommation la plus élevée, affichant une augmentation significative par rapport aux 6,53 S-DDD$_{ptpd}$ de 2022. Le Mexique a observé l'augmentation la plus importante, la consommation étant passée de 0,28 S-DDD$_{ptpd}$ en 2022 à 9,30 S-DDD$_{ptpd}$ en 2023. L'Uruguay (8,05 S-DDD$_{ptpd}$), malgré une baisse par rapport aux 14,08 S-DDD$_{ptpd}$, est resté parmi les pays où la consommation déclarée a été la plus élevée. La consommation au Chili est passée de 3,07 S-DDD$_{ptpd}$ à 7,77 S-DDD$_{ptpd}$. Entre 2022 et 2023, le Costa Rica a également signalé une hausse de la consommation (de 4,89 S-DDD$_{ptpd}$ à 7,22 S-DDD$_{ptpd}$), alors que l'Espagne a signalé une baisse (de 8,12 S-DDD$_{ptpd}$ à 3,73 S-DDD$_{ptpd}$), et le Portugal une hausse (de 2,38 S-DDD$_{ptpd}$ à 5,90 S-DDD$_{ptpd}$).

Alprazolam

66. L'alprazolam, tranquillisant à action brève utilisé dans la prise en charge à court terme des troubles anxieux, est l'une des benzodiazépines le plus fréquemment prescrites dans le monde. En 2023, la fabrication mondiale de cette substance a atteint le niveau record de 15,5 tonnes, contre 12,8 tonnes en 2022. L'Inde a considérablement augmenté sa fabrication, passant de 6,9 tonnes en 2022 à 10,8 tonnes en 2023. Les États-Unis ont déclaré une baisse de la fabrication, de 2,7 tonnes en 2022 à 2,1 tonnes en 2023. L'Italie a déclaré une fabrication totale de 1,7 tonne, la Chine de 513 kg et l'Australie de 201 kg, des quantités moindres étant signalées par quelques autres pays. Les stocks mondiaux d'alprazolam ont légèrement diminué, passant de 7,8 tonnes en 2022 à 7,4 tonnes en 2023, les États-Unis (2,3 tonnes), l'Italie (1,2 tonne), l'Inde (797 kg) et la Chine (745 kg) en détenant les plus importants.

67. Le volume total d'alprazolam importé dans le monde a fortement augmenté en 2023, atteignant 14,9 tonnes, contre 10,1 tonnes en 2022. Au total, 139 pays et territoires ont déclaré des importations en 2023. Israël a connu une hausse significative de ses importations, qui ont atteint 5,2 tonnes, soit une augmentation considérable par rapport aux 8 kg déclarés en 2022, ce qui en fait le plus gros importateur en 2023. Les États-Unis ont suivi avec 1,5 tonne, soit une légère augmentation par rapport à 2022 (1,3 tonne). L'Italie a également fait état d'une augmentation, avec 1,3 tonne importée, contre 664 kg en 2022. Le Brésil a importé 820 kg, contre 1,39 tonne en 2022. La Suisse et l'Irlande ont également enregistré des baisses, avec des importations totales de 504 kg et 399 kg, respectivement. De plus petites quantités ont été importées par divers autres pays.

68. En 2023, 85 pays et territoires ont communiqué des données sur la consommation d'alprazolam. Parmi les pays et territoires déclarants, 11 ont rendu compte de taux supérieurs à 10 S-DDD$_{ptpd}$ et 26 de taux compris entre 2 S-DDD$_{ptpd}$ et 10 S-DDD$_{ptpd}$. Parmi les premiers, la Hongrie (51,02 S-DDD$_{ptpd}$), l'Australie (29,54 S-DDD$_{ptpd}$), le Portugal (26,23 S-DDD$_{ptpd}$), l'Espagne (21,24 S-DDD$_{ptpd}$) et le Monténégro (20,73 S-DDD$_{ptpd}$) en ont été les cinq plus gros consommateurs cette année-là.

Lorazépam

69. La quantité de lorazépam fabriquée au niveau mondial a augmenté entre 2022 et 2023, passant de 8,6 tonnes à 10,2 tonnes. Cette croissance a été principalement observée en Inde, où la fabrication est passée de 1,8 tonne en 2022 à 3,1 tonnes en 2023, et par l'Allemagne, qui a connu une augmentation notable de 954 kg en 2022 à

2,3 tonnes en 2023. En revanche, l'Italie, tout en restant le plus gros fabricant, a enregistré une baisse de 5,4 tonnes en 2022 à 4,3 tonnes en 2023. La Chine, le Costa Rica et les États-Unis en ont fabriqué en plus petites quantités. Les stocks détenus par les fabricants sont passées de 6,9 tonnes en 2022 à 8,8 tonnes en 2023. C'est l'Allemagne qui détenait les plus gros stocks, avec 2,6 tonnes, suivie de l'Italie (1 tonne), du Royaume des Pays-Bas (987 kg) et du Canada (911 kg). De plus petites quantités étaient détenues par 35 autres pays.

70. En 2023, les importations mondiales de lorazépam ont encore chuté pour s'établir à 8,5 tonnes, poursuivant leur tendance à la baisse par rapport aux 8,6 tonnes de 2022 et aux 11,5 tonnes en 2020. L'Espagne a été le plus gros importateur en 2023, avec 1,2 tonne, suivie des États-Unis (1,2 tonne), de l'Irlande (741 kg), du Canada (686 kg) et de l'Allemagne (657 kg). Les exportations mondiales de lorazépam ont suivi une tendance identique, atteignant 9 tonnes en 2023, contre 9,6 tonnes en 2022. En 2023, l'Italie a été une fois de plus le plus gros exportateur de lorazépam, avec 4,5 tonnes. L'Allemagne et l'Inde ont également été des exportateurs importants, avec respectivement 1,6 tonne et 1,3 tonne. Ces trois pays et territoires ont été les seuls à exporter plus d'une tonne de lorazépam en 2023.

71. En 2023, 81 pays et territoires ont déclaré une consommation de lorazépam, contre 70 en 2022. Comme les années précédentes, le Portugal a déclaré le niveau de consommation de lorazépam le plus élevé, avec 34,82 S-DDD_{ptpd}, suivi de l'Espagne (26,92 S-DDD_{ptpd}), du Monténégro (14,13 S-DDD_{ptpd}), de la Belgique (12,92 S-DDD_{ptpd}) et de Malte (11,98 S-DDD_{ptpd}). En outre, 21 autres pays ont déclaré des niveaux de consommation compris entre 2 et 10 S-DDD_{ptpd}. Les autres pays et territoires ont déclaré des niveaux de consommation inférieurs à 2 S-DDD_{ptpd}.

Bromazépam

72. La fabrication de bromazépam a culminé à 15,2 tonnes en 2022 avant de tomber à 9,0 tonnes en 2023, revenant ainsi à des niveaux plus généralement observés les années précédentes. Le chiffre record de 2022 est dû à la Suisse, qui a déclaré 5,9 tonnes après avoir déclaré une fabrication nulle en 2021. En 2023, la Suisse a de nouveau déclaré une fabrication nulle. L'Italie est restée le plus gros fabricant de cette substance, avec 6,2 tonnes. Les autres principaux fabricants étaient l'Inde (1,7 tonne) et le Brésil (1,1 tonne). En 2023, les stocks mondiaux de bromazépam sont passés à 8,8 tonnes, après un record de 11,6 tonnes en 2022. La Suisse a considérablement réduit ses stocks, qui sont passés de 5,5 tonnes en 2022 à 1,7 tonne en 2023. L'Italie a augmenté ses stocks de 1,7 tonne en 2022 à 2,5 tonnes en 2023, tandis que la France a vu les siens diminuer de 1,5 tonne à 1,2 tonne. Le Brésil a maintenu des niveaux de stocks relativement stables, déclarant 1,2 tonne, soit une légère baisse par rapport à la quantité de 1,3 tonne déclarée en 2022.

73. En 2023, les importations mondiales de bromazépam ont augmenté pour atteindre 15,9 tonnes, contre 13,1 tonnes en 2022, sous l'effet d'une hausse significative des importations de l'Allemagne, qui ont plus que doublé, passant de 1,9 tonne en 2022 à 4,5 tonnes en 2023. La Serbie, quant à elle, a vu ses importations diminuer de 1,2 tonne à 893 kg. En 2023, les autres principaux importateurs étaient le Pakistan (1,7 tonne), la France (1,6 tonne) et l'Italie (837 kg). Les exportations totales de bromazépam ont augmenté de 13,7 tonnes en 2022 à 16,3 tonnes en 2023. Les principaux exportateurs en 2023 étaient l'Italie (5,8 tonnes), la Suisse (4,4 tonnes), l'Allemagne (3,2 tonnes) et l'Inde (1,7 tonne).

74. Les plus gros consommateurs de bromazépam en 2023 étaient le Monténégro (15,47 S-DDD_{ptpd}) et la Bosnie-Herzégovine (15,38 S-DDD_{ptpd}). Les autres pays ayant déclaré des niveaux de consommation supérieurs à 4 S-DDD_{ptpd} pour l'année sont la France, avec 5,43 S-DDD_{ptpd}, et la Lituanie, où la consommation est restée stable à 4,75 S-DDD_{ptpd}.

Clobazam

75. La quantité de clobazam fabriquée au niveau mondial a diminué entre 2022 et 2023, passant de 12,3 tonnes à 8,7 tonnes. Cette baisse est principalement due à l'absence de déclaration de fabrication par la France, alors qu'elle avait déclaré 4,5 tonnes l'année précédente. En 2023, l'Inde a été le premier fabricant mondial avec 6,6 tonnes, suivie de l'Allemagne, avec 1,9 tonne. Les États-Unis, l'Italie et le Pérou ont fait état de quantités nettement inférieures.

76. Les importations mondiales de clobazam ont légèrement diminué, passant à 7,4 tonnes en 2023, après des niveaux relativement stables de 7,5 tonnes en 2022 et de 7,9 tonnes en 2021. L'Inde en a été le plus gros importateur en 2023, avec 1,2 tonne, suivie de la France (999 kg), des États-Unis (792 kg), du Brésil (766 kg) et de l'Indonésie (447 kg). Les exportations mondiales ont également peu évolué par rapport à 2022, s'établissant à 8,2 tonnes. Les seuls pays à exporter de grosses quantités ont été la France (3,4 tonnes), l'Inde (2,5 tonnes) et l'Allemagne (1,5 tonne).

77. En 2023, 66 pays et territoires ont déclaré une consommation de clobazam, contre 55 en 2022. Le Portugal et la Nouvelle-Zélande ont affiché les taux les plus élevés, avec respectivement 1,11 S-DDD_{ptpd} et 1,10 S-DDD_{ptpd}. L'Uruguay suit avec 0,89 S-DDD_{ptpd}, tandis que le Canada (0,83 S-DDD_{ptpd}) et la France (0,73 S-DDD_{ptpd}) enregistrent également des niveaux de consommation substantiels.

Chlordiazépoxide

78. La quantité de chlordiazépoxide fabriquée au niveau mondial a connu de fortes fluctuations ces dernières années. Après avoir augmenté jusqu'à 24,2 tonnes en 2021 et atteint un pic de 25,5 tonnes en 2022, la fabrication mondiale a diminué, pour atteindre 22,8 tonnes en 2023, principalement en raison de réductions en Italie et en Inde. La fabrication déclarée par l'Italie est passée de 13,6 tonnes en 2022 à 12,2 tonnes en 2023, et celle de l'Inde de 11,3 tonnes en 2022 à 9,6 tonnes en 2023. Dans le même temps, la fabrication de chlordiazépoxide en Chine a atteint 978 kg en 2023, contre 600 kg en 2022. Les stocks de chlordiazépoxide détenus par les fabricants ont augmenté entre 2022 et 2023, passant de 9,8 tonnes à 10,7 tonnes, et ils étaient détenus par 31 pays, pour la majorité l'Italie (4,9 tonnes), l'Inde (1,4 tonne), les États-Unis (807 kg) et la Chine (717 kg).

79. Les importations mondiales de chlordiazépoxide ont fluctué autour de 13 tonnes depuis 2020. Après un record de 14,1 tonnes en 2020, les importations ont chuté à 13,9 tonnes en 2022 et 13 tonnes en 2023. La Suisse est restée le principal importateur de cette substance en 2023, avec 6,2 tonnes, suivie du Pakistan et de l'Égypte, qui en ont importé chacun un peu plus de 1,2 tonne. L'Italie (12,4 tonnes), la Suisse (6,1 tonnes) et l'Inde (1,5 tonne) ont représenté plus de 96 % de toutes les exportations de chlordiazépoxide en 2023.

80. En 2023, 50 pays et territoires ont déclaré une consommation de chlordiazépoxide. L'Islande a déclaré le niveau de consommation le plus élevé, avec 1,29 S-DDD_{ptpd}, suivie de près par le Portugal avec 1,20 S-DDD_{ptpd}. D'autres niveaux de consommation importants ont été signalés par le Liban (0,76 S-DDD_{ptpd}), le Chili (0,70 S-DDD_{ptpd}) et l'Albanie (0,63 S-DDD_{ptpd}).

Oxazépam

81. La fabrication mondiale d'oxazépam suit une tendance à la baisse depuis le record de 27,5 tonnes atteint en 2019. Elle est passée à 22,8 tonnes en 2020 et 22,7 tonnes en 2021, puis a continué à diminuer pour atteindre 19,9 tonnes en 2022 et 18,8 tonnes en 2023. Cette tendance à la baisse est imputable à la diminution de la production en Italie, le principal fabricant, qui a déclaré 27,3 tonnes en 2019 et 15,3 tonnes en 2023. La fabrication en Inde, qui a connu des fluctuations ces dernières années, est tombée à 1,25 tonne en 2023. Dans le même temps, la Chine, qui a commencé à fabriquer des quantités significatives en 2021, a déclaré 2,2 tonnes en 2023. Les stocks d'oxazépam détenus par les fabricants ont eux aussi diminué depuis le pic de 32,7 tonnes atteint en 2020, tombant à 21,4 tonnes en 2022 et à 16,7 tonnes en 2023. Les stocks d'oxazépam des fabricants étaient détenus par 24 pays, pour la majorité en France (7 tonnes), en Italie (3,2 tonnes), en Autriche (995 kg) et au Canada (931 kg).

82. Les importations mondiales d'oxazépam ont diminué depuis 2019, année où elles ont atteint un pic de 30,5 tonnes. Les importations ont chuté à 26,9 tonnes en 2020, puis à 19,9 tonnes en 2022 et 2023. La France a été le premier importateur d'oxazépam, avec 9,7 tonnes en 2023, contre 8,3 tonnes en 2022. Elle était suivie par l'Allemagne, avec 1,8 tonne, soit une légère augmentation par rapport à l'année précédente (1,7 tonne). La Pologne a également augmenté ses importations, à 1,6 tonne, et l'Afrique du Sud a importé 1,2 tonne en 2023. L'Italie (16,4 tonnes), l'Allemagne (1,4 tonne), la Pologne (979 kg) et l'Inde (959 kg) représentaient 97 % de toutes les exportations d'oxazépam en 2023.

Français

83. En 2023, 34 pays ont déclaré une consommation d'oxazépam. La France a déclaré le niveau de consommation d'oxazépam le plus élevé, avec 9,24 S-DDD_{ptpd}, suivie de l'Islande (5,63 S-DDD_{ptpd}), de la Norvège (4,66 S-DDD_{ptpd}), de la Finlande (4,38 S-DDD_{ptpd}), de l'Autriche (3,53 S-DDD_{ptpd}), du Royaume des Pays-Bas (3,30 S-DDD_{ptpd}), du Portugal (2,29 S-DDD_{ptpd}), de la Suède (2,16 S-DDD_{ptpd}) et de la Suisse (2,01 S-DDD_{ptpd}).

Autres benzodiazépines présentes en quantité non négligeable sur le marché licite

84. L'alprazolam, le bromazépam, le chlordiazépoxide, le clobazam, le clonazépam, le diazépam, le lorazépam, le midazolam et l'oxazépam représentent 90 % des benzodiazépines fabriquées licitement et présentes en quantité non négligeable sur le marché licite, les 10 % restants correspondant à sept autres substances : le nitrazépam, le clorazépate, le triazolam, le témazépam, le flunitrazépam, le prazépam et le flurazépam.

Nitrazépam

85. La fabrication de nitrazépam a légèrement augmenté, passant de 2,7 tonnes l'année précédente à environ 2,9 tonnes en 2023. En 2023, l'Italie en était le principal fabricant, avec 1,5 tonne, suivie de près par l'Inde, qui a déclaré une fabrication totale de 1,4 tonne. Les stocks ont poursuivi leur tendance à la baisse, passant de 1,9 tonne en 2022 à 1,4 tonne en 2023. En 2023, l'Italie en détenait les plus gros stocks (292 kg) devant la France (202 kg), le reste étant réparti entre 22 autres pays. Sur le plan mondial, les importations ont augmenté, passant de 1,5 tonne en 2022 à 2 tonnes en 2023. De même, les exportations sont passées de 1,6 tonne à 2 tonnes. Cette année-là, 36 pays ont déclaré une consommation de nitrazépam, Malte affichant le niveau de consommation le plus élevé (1,98 S-DDD_{ptpd}).

Clorazépate

86. La fabrication mondiale de clorazépate, qui était en baisse depuis 2019, a connu une tendance inverse en 2023, atteignant 1,5 tonne, contre 794 kg en 2022. L'Italie a été le principal fabricant de la substance en 2023. Les stocks ont augmenté de manière significative, passant de 1,5 tonne en 2022 à 6,6 tonnes en 2023. Les importations mondiales de clorazépate ont également fortement augmenté, passant de 4,4 tonnes en 2022 à 8,3 tonnes en 2023. Quant aux exportations mondiales, elles ont légèrement diminué, s'établissant à 4,2 tonnes. En 2023, 25 pays ont déclaré une consommation de clorazépate, l'Espagne affichant le niveau de consommation le plus élevé (3,97 S-DDD_{ptpd}).

Triazolam

87. Après un pic à 1,1 tonne en 2021, la fabrication mondiale de triazolam est tombée à 252 kg en 2022, puis à 58 kg en 2023, soit le deuxième niveau le plus bas depuis que la substance a été placée sous contrôle international. Cette baisse est due à une diminution importante de la fabrication aux États-Unis et au fait qu'aucune fabrication n'a été déclarée par l'Italie. En 2023, trois pays ont assuré la totalité de la fabrication de cette substance : les États-Unis (31 kg), l'Inde (22 kg) et la République de Corée (5 kg). Les stocks ont diminué de 75 kg pour atteindre 308 kg en 2023, la majorité étant détenue par les États-Unis (156 kg), l'Italie (72 kg) et l'Irlande (38 kg). Les importations et les exportations de triazolam ont poursuivi leur tendance à la baisse en 2023. Les importations et les exportations sont tombées à 123 kg, en recul par rapport à 2022, année pendant laquelle les deux s'élevaient à environ 170 kg. En 2023, 26 pays ont déclaré une consommation de triazolam, l'Autriche affichant le niveau de consommation le plus élevé (5,63 S-DDD_{ptpd}).

Témazépam

88. La fabrication de témazépam a légèrement rebondi en 2023, passant à 6,9 tonnes après avoir atteint son niveau le plus bas en 10 ans, à savoir 5,4 tonnes en 2022. Toutefois, le total pour 2023 est resté bien en deçà des 11,6 tonnes déclarées en 2021. L'Italie est à nouveau le plus gros fabricant de cette substance en 2023, avec

6,3 tonnes. L'Inde suit avec 181 kg, tandis que l'Australie et la Pologne ont déclaré des quantités moindres, à savoir 200 kg et 131 kg, respectivement. En 2023, les stocks de témazépam sont tombés à 8,3 tonnes, poursuivant leur tendance à la baisse amorcée les années précédentes, la majorité étant détenue par l'Italie (2,5 tonnes), l'Inde et le Canada, qui ont tous deux déclaré environ 1 tonne. Les importations totales déclarées de témazépam ont légèrement augmenté, passant de 7,7 tonnes en 2022 à 8,2 tonnes en 2023. De même, les exportations totales ont augmenté, passant de 7,5 tonnes en 2022 à 8,5 tonnes en 2023. Sur les 19 pays qui ont communiqué des données, le Royaume des Pays-Bas a déclaré le niveau de consommation le plus élevé de cette substance (4,08 S-DDD_{ptpd}).

Flunitrazépam

89. La quantité de flunitrazépam fabriquée a considérablement fluctué ces dernières années, passant de 2,2 tonnes en 2020 à 36 kg en 2021, avant de remonter à 182 kg en 2022 et à 544 kg en 2023. L'Italie en a été le plus gros fabricant en 2023 avec 240 kg, suivie du Japon (165 kg) et de l'Inde (138 kg). Les stocks sont passés de 614 kg en 2023 contre 979 kg en 2022, l'Italie en détenant la majorité (193 kg). Les importations de cette substance sont passées de 1,8 tonne en 2020 à 432 kg en 2022, avant de remonter à 809 kg en 2023. De même, les exportations mondiales sont passées de 1,9 tonne en 2020 à 530 kg en 2022, puis à 945 kg en 2023. En 2022, c'est l'Uruguay qui en a déclaré la consommation la plus élevée, celle-ci s'établissant à 29,12 S-DDD_{ptpd}, soit presque le double qu'en 2022. Dix-neuf autres pays ont déclaré en détenir, en petites quantités.

Prazépam

90. La fabrication de prazépam a considérablement augmenté en 2023, atteignant 3,9 tonnes, soit plus du double des 1,7 tonnes déclarées en 2022, poursuivant ainsi la reprise après le creux de 850 kg atteint en 2020. L'Italie en a été l'unique fabricant de la substance en 2023. Les stocks de prazépam ont augmenté pour atteindre 3,4 tonnes en 2023, après une baisse progressive de 7,1 tonnes en 2018 à 2,4 tonnes en 2022. Les stocks étaient détenus par 12 pays. Les importations de prazépam ont augmenté pour atteindre 4 tonnes en 2023, contre 3,4 tonnes l'année précédente. De même, les exportations ont légèrement reculé, s'établissant à 3,7 tonnes en 2023 contre 3,5 tonnes en 2022. En 2023, seuls 13 pays ont déclaré une consommation de cette substance, la quantité la plus élevée ayant été déclarée par la France (2,07 S-DDD_{ptpd}).

Flurazépam

91. La fabrication mondiale de flurazépam a rebondi à 2,8 tonnes en 2023, après une chute importante en 2022, avec seulement 1,3 tonne fabriquée, contre 3,4 tonnes en 2021. L'augmentation est principalement due à une reprise en Italie, qui a déclaré avoir fabriqué 2 tonnes en 2023 après seulement 880 kg en 2022. La totalité des stocks détenus en 2023 s'élevaient à 2,3 tonnes, l'Italie détenant la plus grosse quantité (1 tonne). Les importations ont augmenté, passant de 1,5 tonne en 2022 à 1,7 tonne en 2023. De même, les exportations ont légèrement augmenté, s'établissant à 2,1 tonnes en 2023 contre 1,7 tonne en 2022. En 2023, 17 pays ont déclaré une consommation de cette substance, la quantité la plus élevée ayant été déclarée par l'Espagne (0,92 S-DDD_{ptpd}).

Barbituriques

92. En 2023, seuls trois barbituriques sous contrôle international étaient présents en quantité non négligeable sur le marché licite (voir tableau 10). La fabrication de pentobarbital et de barbital a augmenté, rompant avec la tendance à la baisse des dernières décennies. Dans le même temps, la fabrication de phénobarbital a poursuivi sa tendance à la hausse, augmentant de près de 10 tonnes par rapport à l'année précédente. L'amobarbital et le butalbital, qui ne figurent pas dans le tableau 10, sont toujours fabriqués et commercialisés en quantités relativement importantes.

Français

Tableau 10. Barbituriques présents en quantité non négligeable sur le marché licite : fabrication et importations mondiales totales (classement en fonction du nombre de pays et territoires importateurs), 2023

Substance	*S-DDD (en mg)*	*Quantité fabriquée (en kg)*	*Importations (en kg)*	*Nombre de pays et territoires importateurs*
Phénobarbital	100	374 079,15	208 219,59	158
Pentobarbital	100	58 630,12	61 852,59	68
Barbital	500	58 313,31	2 965,38	22

Phénobarbital

93. En termes de poids brut, le phénobarbital est la substance psychotrope soumise à contrôle international la plus fabriquée depuis 2012. En 2023, il a été déclaré au total une quantité fabriquée de 374 tonnes, soit une légère hausse par rapport aux 364,3 tonnes déclarées en 2022. Malgré une baisse de 46,8 tonnes par rapport à l'année précédente, la Chine est restée le plus gros fabricant de phénobarbital, dont elle a produit 174,9 tonnes en 2023. L'Inde, l'autre grand fabricant de cette substance, a déclaré un total de 130,9 tonnes en 2023, soit 31 tonnes de plus que l'année précédente. Les seuls autres pays à déclarer en avoir fabriqué des quantités importantes en 2023 ont été la Hongrie (42,2 tonnes) et la Fédération de Russie (24,3 tonnes).

94. Les stocks de phénobarbital détenus par les fabricants ont augmenté de 62,7 tonnes entre 2022 et 2023, passant de 182,4 tonnes à 245,1 tonnes. Les stocks les plus importants étaient détenus par la Chine (67,9 tonnes), la Fédération de Russie (49,4 tonnes), la Hongrie (33,0 tonnes) et le Brésil (26,0 tonnes). En outre, 12 pays ont déclaré des stocks compris entre 1 et 10,8 tonnes, et 33 autres des stocks inférieurs à 1 tonne.

95. En 2023, 158 pays et territoires ont déclaré des importations de phénobarbital, ce qui en fait l'une des substances psychotropes placées sous contrôle international les plus échangées. En 2023, le volume total des importations mondiales de cette substance a ainsi atteint 208,2 tonnes, ce qui représente une légère diminution par rapport aux 213 tonnes de 2022. Le pays qui en a importé la plus grosse quantité était le Brésil (41,2 tonnes), suivi de la Fédération de Russie (23,0 tonnes), des États-Unis (19 tonnes), de la Suisse (10,0 tonnes) et du Danemark (8,9 tonnes). Vingt-deux autres pays en ont déclaré des importations allant de 1 tonne à 6,8 tonnes. Les importations déclarées par les autres pays et territoires varient considérablement, allant de quelques dizaines de grammes à plusieurs centaines de kilogrammes.

Figure 13. Phénobarbital : nombre de pays et territoires ayant déclaré la consommation de cette substance, par région (2019-2023)

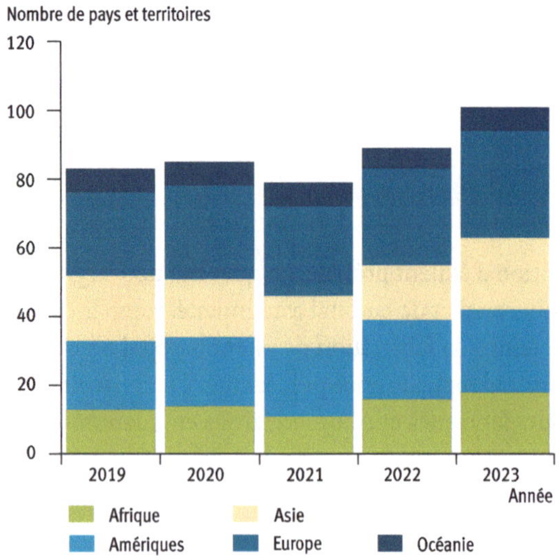

96. Les exportations totales de phénobarbital ont considérablement diminué, passant de 226,8 tonnes en 2022 à 199,8 tonnes en 2023, en partie en raison d'une réduction significative des exportations de la Chine, deuxième exportateur en 2023. Les exportations de phénobarbital du pays ont chuté de 86,1 tonnes en 2022 à 59,8 tonnes en 2023. Les autres principaux exportateurs de cette substance en 2023 étaient l'Inde (79 tonnes), la Hongrie (20,7 tonnes), la Suisse (9,7 tonnes), le Danemark (9,1 tonnes), l'Allemagne (5,2 tonnes), la Croatie (3,1 tonnes), la France (2,7 tonnes), le Royaume des Pays-Bas (2,4 tonnes), la Roumanie (2,3 tonnes) et le Kenya (1,5 tonne).

97. Le nombre de pays et territoires ayant déclaré une consommation de phénobarbital a augmenté, passant de 89 en 2022 à 101 en 2023. La figure 13 présente une comparaison par région du nombre de pays et territoires ayant communiqué des données à ce sujet entre 2019 et 2023. Les régions dans lesquelles ils ont

été le plus nombreux à le faire étaient les Amériques et l'Europe. En valeur absolue, c'est en Océanie qu'ils ont été le moins nombreux à le faire. En 2023, cinq nouveaux pays et territoires d'Asie ont communiqué des données, alors que le nombre correspondant de pays d'Afrique n'a que légèrement augmenté.

98. Parmi les pays et territoires ayant fourni des données, c'est le Brésil qui a indiqué le plus haut niveau de consommation de cette substance (4,96 S-DDD_{ptpd}), niveau légèrement supérieur à celui de l'année précédente (4,95 S-DDD_{ptpd}). En Europe, Saint-Marin (2,17 S-DDD_{ptpd}) a été le plus gros consommateur, suivi de la France (1,28 S-DDD_{ptpd}) et du Monténégro (1,24 S-DDD_{ptpd}). En Afrique, les Seychelles en ont déclaré le plus (4,81 S-DDD_{ptpd}), tandis que le Burkina Faso en a déclaré le moins (0,01 S-DDD_{ptpd}). Dans les Amériques, on observe également une grande hétérogénéité intrarégionale ; comme indiqué plus haut, le Brésil a déclaré la consommation la plus élevée de cette substance (4,96 S-DDD_{ptpd}) et Cuba la plus basse (moins de 0,03 S-DDD_{ptpd}). En Asie, les quantités consommées dans les pays et territoires ayant communiqué des données ont également nettement varié : ainsi, la Chine a déclaré la consommation la plus élevée (2,48 S-DDD_{ptpd}) et l'Iraq la plus faible (0,003 S-DDD_{ptpd}). En Océanie, sept pays et territoires ont communiqué des données sur la consommation de phénobarbital, et c'est l'Australie qui en a déclaré la quantité la plus élevée (0,85 S-DDD_{ptpd}).

99. Des informations plus détaillées concernant la consommation de phénobarbital sont disponibles sur le site Web de l'OICS.

Pentobarbital

100. Une nouvelle fois, les États-Unis et l'Allemagne ont été les principaux fabricants de pentobarbital en 2023, puisqu'ils ont déclaré en avoir fabriqué respectivement 33,6 tonnes et 24,6 tonnes. Le Japon a fait état d'une augmentation significative de la fabrication de cette substance, qui est passée de 0,5 kg (2022) à 353 kg (2023). Au total, 58,6 tonnes de pentobarbital ont été fabriquées en 2023, ce qui représente une légère augmentation par rapport aux 56,0 tonnes déclarées en 2022. En 2023, les quantités de cette substance fabriquées en Allemagne et aux États-Unis sont restées pratiquement inchangées par rapport à l'année précédente. L'Inde et la Suisse ont également signalé la fabrication de cette substance, mais dans des quantités de quelques grammes chacune.

101. Les stocks détenus par les fabricants sont passées de 43,0 tonnes en 2022 à 55,6 tonnes en 2023. Les États-Unis en détenaient quelques 16,8 tonnes et l'Allemagne 16,7 tonnes, devant le Royaume des Pays-Bas (8 tonnes), le Danemark (3,4 tonnes), la France (3,3 tonnes), l'Autriche (2,4 tonnes), la Suisse et le Royaume-Uni (1,2 tonne chacun). Seize autres pays ont déclaré des stocks de cette substance, chacun n'en détenant pas plus de quelques centaines de kilogrammes.

102. En 2023, le Royaume des Pays-Bas a été le principal pays importateur de pentobarbital, avec 16,5 tonnes, soit 4,7 tonnes de plus qu'en 2022 (11,8 tonnes). L'essentiel de ses importations était destiné à la réexportation. Les importations de pentobarbital déclarées par les autres pays sont restées largement inchangées par rapport aux années précédentes ; les autres principaux importateurs étaient le Danemark (7,0 tonnes) et l'Allemagne (6,6 tonnes). Huit autres pays ont déclaré en avoir importé au moins une tonne. Dix-huit autres pays ont déclaré en avoir importé entre 100 kg et 1 tonne, les quantités déclarées par les autres pays variant de quelques grammes à plusieurs dizaines de kilogrammes.

103. Sur le plan mondial, les exportations ont également augmenté, passant de 41,5 tonnes en 2022 à 47,5 tonnes en 2023. L'Allemagne, qui est l'un des principaux pays fabricant de pentobarbital, en est également le premier exportateur avec 22,3 tonnes, ce qui est légèrement inférieur au 23,0 tonnes déclarées en 2022. Le Royaume des Pays-Bas en a été le deuxième exportateur, puisqu'il en a déclaré 11,8 tonnes, soit un peu moins que les années précédentes. Le Danemark et l'Autriche ont déclaré des exportations de plus de 5,1 tonnes et 3,4 tonnes, respectivement.

104. Pour 2023, 44 pays et territoires au total ont communiqué des données sur la consommation de pentobarbital, soit plus qu'en 2022 (38 pays). Le Luxembourg en a déclaré la consommation la plus élevée, s'établissant à 4,14 S-DDD_{ptpd}, légèrement inférieure à celle de 2022 (4,92 S-DDD_{ptpd}). Les seuls autres pays à en avoir déclaré une consommation supérieure à 3 S-DDD_{ptpd} ont été le Danemark et l'Australie.

Barbital

105. La fabrication mondiale de barbital est passée de 48,6 tonnes en 2022 à 58,3 tonnes en 2023, dépassant le précédent record de 57,9 tonnes enregistré en 2019. La Chine en est restée le principal fabricant, puisqu'elle en a déclaré 36,8 tonnes en 2023, soit plus qu'en 2022 (30,6 tonnes). Les seuls autres pays à déclarer en avoir fabriqué en 2023 ont été l'Inde (20,0 tonnes), l'Allemagne (1,1 tonne) et le Japon (341 kg). Les quantités fabriquées dans ces pays n'ont pas beaucoup changé par rapport à l'année précédente, sauf en Inde, qui a déclaré 20 tonnes contre 13 tonnes l'année précédente. Les stocks de barbital des fabricants ont atteint 46,8 tonnes en 2023, ce qui représente une augmentation significative par rapport aux 29,1 tonnes déclarées en 2022. La Chine en détenait 40,7 tonnes, soit près de 87 % des stocks mondiaux et presque le double du chiffre déclaré pour 2022, la majeure partie de la quantité restante étant détenue par l'Allemagne (4,3 tonnes) et la France (812 kg).

106. Le commerce du barbital a été quelque peu limité, seuls 22 pays et territoires en ayant déclaré des importations. Les importations totales pour 2023 se sont élevées à un peu moins de 3 tonnes, soit 234 kg de plus que les 2,7 tonnes déclarées pour 2022. En 2023, le plus gros importateur de barbital était les États-Unis (1,2 tonne), devant la France (742,4 kg), la Thaïlande (712,7 kg), la Suisse (166,8 kg) et le Royaume-Uni (97,5 kg). Les exportations totales de cette substance ont diminué de seulement 26 kg pour s'établir à 2,6 tonnes en 2023, l'Allemagne (1,9 tonne) en représentant la plus grosse part. Les seuls autres pays à déclarer en avoir exporté des quantités non négligeables ont été le Japon (357,6 kg) et la Suisse (187,5 kg).

107. En ce qui concerne la consommation de barbital, on ne dispose de données que pour quelques pays. En 2023, sur les 16 pays ayant communiqué des données, tous, à l'exception de la Chine (0,06 $\text{S-DDD}_{\text{ptpd}}$), en ont déclaré une consommation inférieure à 0,01 $\text{S-DDD}_{\text{ptpd}}$.

Autres sédatifs hypnotiques

108. Des huit sédatifs hypnotiques qui ne sont ni des benzodiazépines ni des barbituriques, seuls deux font actuellement l'objet d'un commerce licite : l'acide *gamma*-hydroxybutyrique (GHB) et le zolpidem. Les statistiques relatives au GHB doivent être interprétées avec prudence car la S-DDD de cette substance est actuellement de 7 500 mg, soit largement supérieure à celle de toute autre substance psychotrope placée sous contrôle international. La plupart des substances placées sous contrôle en vertu de la Convention de 1971 ayant des S-DDD comprises entre 1 et 200 mg, les chiffres bruts de la fabrication et du commerce de GHB peuvent donner à penser que cette substance est très présente sur le marché. En réalité, la valeur élevée de la S-DDD du GHB s'explique par le fait que, comparativement à d'autres substances, il faut la fabriquer en beaucoup plus grosses quantités — 10 voire 100 fois plus — pour obtenir des niveaux de dosage équivalents. Cette disproportion est illustrée par le tableau 11, où le poids de base correspondant à une dose quotidienne déterminée à des fins statistiques est 750 fois plus élevé pour le GHB que pour le zolpidem.

Tableau 11. Autres sédatifs hypnotiques présents en quantité non négligeable sur le marché licite : quantités totales fabriquées à l'échelle mondiale et nombre de pays et territoires importateurs (classés en fonction de la quantité fabriquée en S-DDD) (2023)

Substance	*S-DDD (en mg)*	*Quantité fabriquée (en kg)*	*Quantité fabriquée (en millions de S-DDD)*	*Nombre de pays et territoires importateurs*
Zolpidem	10	40 740,39	4 074,04	118
Acide *gamma*-hydroxybutyrique	7 500	57 789,12	7,71	43

Acide *gamma*-hydroxybutyrique

109. Compte tenu de sa valeur élevée en S-DDD, le GHB doit être fabriqué en bien plus grandes quantités pour pouvoir répondre à la demande mondiale à des fins médicales et scientifiques, même s'il ne fait pas l'objet d'un commerce aussi important que d'autres substances placées sous contrôle.

110. Pour 2023, on a déclaré la fabrication de 57,8 tonnes de GHB, ce qui représente une hausse considérable par rapport aux 51,9 tonnes déclarées pour 2022. Cette augmentation s'explique principalement par le fait que

l'Irlande, qui avait déclaré n'en avoir pas fabriqué du tout en 2021, en a repris la fabrication en 2022 et en 2023. En 2023, l'Irlande (26,2 tonnes) en a été le principal fabricant, suivie des États-Unis (15,0 tonnes) et de l'Inde (9,8 tonnes). Les stocks détenus par les fabricants ont nettement augmenté, passant de 119,7 tonnes en 2022 à 217,0 tonnes en 2023. Le principal détenteur de stocks était l'Irlande, qui a déclaré un peu plus de 61,9 tonnes, suivie des États-Unis (20,8 tonnes), de la France (6,5 tonnes), de l'Ukraine (3,5 tonnes), de l'Italie (3,0 tonnes) et de l'Allemagne (2,8 tonnes). La Suisse a déclaré une diminution nette de ses stocks de GHB, qui sont passés de 2,5 tonnes en 2021 à 207,9 kg en 2023, du fait des exportations.

111. En 2023, 43 pays et territoires ont déclaré des importations de GHB, qui s'élevaient au total à 62,9 tonnes, soit une baisse sensible par rapport aux 78,1 tonnes déclarées par 41 pays en 2022. Ce sont les États-Unis qui ont déclaré en avoir importé la plus grosse quantité (35,8 tonnes), suivis de la France (4,6 tonnes), de l'Italie (4,1 tonnes), de la Belgique (4,0 tonnes), de la Lettonie (2,7 tonnes), de la Fédération de Russie (2,0 tonnes) et de l'Espagne (1,7 tonne). Trois autres pays ont déclaré en avoir importé plus d'une tonne, tandis que les autres pays et territoires ont déclaré en avoir importé de plus faibles quantités.

112. Les exportations de GHB ont diminué entre 2022 et 2023, passant de 76,4 tonnes à 63,3 tonnes. Cette baisse est principalement attribuable à des diminutions importantes des exportations de l'Irlande, qui ont reculé de 42,5 tonnes en 2022 à 32,5 tonnes en 2023, mais qui est néanmoins restée le principal exportateur de cette substance. Elle était suivie par les États-Unis (7,1 tonnes), l'Allemagne (6,4 tonnes), l'Inde (4,1 tonnes), la France (4,0 tonnes), la Belgique (3,0 tonnes), la Lettonie (2,6 tonnes) et le Royaume-Uni (1,5 tonne), et cinq autres pays ont déclaré des exportations de GHB comprises entre 100 kg et 1 tonne.

113. En 2023, la consommation de GHB a été déclarée principalement par des pays d'Europe, ainsi que par le Canada et les États-Unis, ce qui confirme la tendance observée ces dernières années. Ce sont les États-Unis qui en ont déclaré la plus forte consommation (0,04 $S\text{-}DDD_{ptpd}$). L'Italie, la Norvège, les Pays-Bas (Royaume des) et la Suède en ont chacun déclaré une consommation de 0,02 $S\text{-}DDD_{ptpd}$. Les autres pays ayant communiqué des données à ce sujet en ont tous déclaré une consommation inférieure à 0,02 $S\text{-}DDD_{ptpd}$.

Français

Zolpidem

114. Le zolpidem est l'une des substances psychotropes placées sous contrôle international les plus échangées. En 2023, 118 pays et territoires en ont déclaré des importations, et sa consommation a été signalée dans toutes les régions du monde.

115. Sa fabrication a légèrement augmenté, passant de 39,1 tonnes en 2022 à 40,7 tonnes en 2023. Comme les années précédentes, l'Inde a été le principal fabricant de cette substance, puisqu'elle en a déclaré 25,8 tonnes, contre 4,6 tonnes en 2022. Elle était suivie par la Tchéquie, qui a déclaré 7,6 tonnes, contre 0,4 tonne en 2022. Le Brésil, qui avait déclaré en avoir fabriqué 4,2 tonnes en 2022, en a déclaré 3,1 tonnes en 2023. Le Japon et l'Argentine ont également été des fabricants importants de zolpidem en 2023, avec 2,6 tonnes et une tonne respectivement. La France, qui avait déclaré 3,5 tonnes fabriquées en 2022, n'a rien déclaré pour 2023.

116. Les stocks mondiaux de zolpidem des fabricants ont presque quintuplé, passant de 18,4 tonnes en 2022 à 87,9 tonnes en 2023. La plus grosse quantité était détenue par la France (16,2 tonnes), suivie par l'Afrique du Sud (6,7 tonnes), le Brésil (4,4 tonnes), l'Inde (3,1 tonnes) et la Tchéquie (3,0 tonnes). De plus petites quantités étaient détenues par 33 autres pays.

117. Les exportations totales de zolpidem ont augmenté de 25,5 tonnes en 2022 à 35,8 tonnes en 2023. Comme les années précédentes, ce sont les États-Unis qui en ont importé la plus grosse quantité (4,9 tonnes), c'est-à-dire moins qu'en 2022 (6,4 tonnes). Les autres principaux importateurs de cette substance ont été le Brésil (3,9 tonnes), l'Espagne (3,0 tonnes), l'Allemagne (2,9 tonnes), le Japon (1,6 tonne), la Pologne (1,6 tonne) et l'Argentine (1,5 tonne). Plusieurs de ces pays en ont importé à des fins de réexportation.

118. Les exportations totales de zolpidem restent relativement stables depuis plusieurs années. En 2023, il en a été déclaré 37,6 tonnes au total, ce qui représente un recul modéré par rapport aux 41,6 tonnes de 2022, qui représentaient elles-mêmes une augmentation par rapport aux 37,3 tonnes déclarées pour 2021. Premier fabricant de zolpidem, l'Inde en a également exporté la plus grosse quantité en 2023 (13,6 tonnes), ce qui est inférieur

Figure 14. Zolpidem : nombre de pays et territoires ayant déclaré la consommation de cette substance, par région (2019-2023)

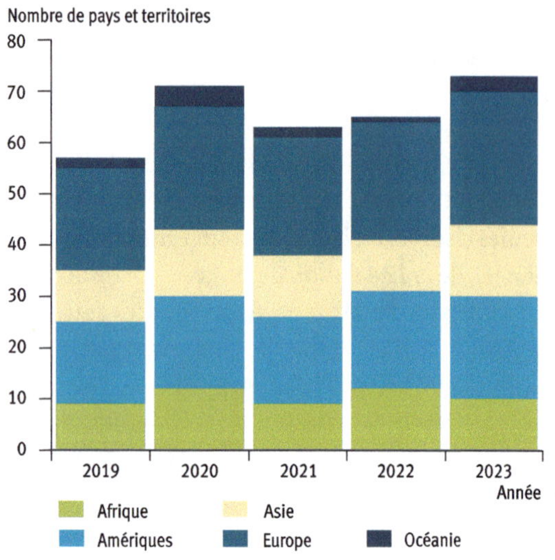

à la quantité déclarée pour 2022 (18,1 tonnes). Les autres principaux exportateurs de cette substance ont été la Tchéquie (7,7 tonnes) et la France (5,4 tonnes). L'Allemagne, l'Espagne, les Pays-Bas (Royaume des) et la Serbie ont chacun déclaré des exportations de 1 tonne à 2 tonnes environ.

119. Au total, huit pays et territoires supplémentaires ont communiqué des données sur la consommation de zolpidem, ce qui fait un total de 73 (voir fig. 14). Au niveau régional, on a observé une augmentation du nombre de déclarations dans toutes les régions. L'Europe est la seule région dans laquelle plus de la moitié des pays et territoires ont fourni des données sur la consommation.

120. En 2023, la Bosnie-Herzégovine a été le pays qui a déclaré le plus haut niveau de consommation de zolpidem au monde (91,03 S-DDD$_{ptpd}$), suivi de la Tchéquie (16,74 S-DDD$_{ptpd}$). Dans l'ensemble, pour les pays et territoires qui ont communiqué des données, la consommation moyenne de zolpidem a été sensiblement plus élevée en Europe que dans les autres régions. En Afrique, le Maroc a déclaré la consommation la plus importante (0,54 S-DDD$_{ptpd}$) et l'Angola la plus faible (0,002 S-DDD$_{ptpd}$). Dans les Amériques, le Brésil en a déclaré la consommation la plus élevée (7,160 S-DDD$_{ptpd}$) et l'Équateur la plus basse (0,01 S-DDD$_{ptpd}$). En Asie, la République de Corée en a déclaré la plus forte consommation (8,96 S-DDD$_{ptpd}$) et les Maldives la plus faible (0,04 S-DDD$_{ptpd}$). En Océanie, l'Australie a déclaré le niveau de consommation le plus élevé (0,97 S-DDD$_{ptpd}$), tandis que les États fédérés de Micronésie ont déclaré le niveau le plus bas (0,002 S-DDD$_{ptpd}$).

Méprobamate

121. Parmi les anxiolytiques placés sous contrôle international présents en quantité non négligeable sur le marché licite, le méprobamate, substance inscrite au Tableau IV de la Convention de 1971, est le seul qui ne soit pas de type benzodiazépine. Bien que cette substance ne fasse l'objet d'échanges qu'entre une douzaine de pays, elle est, en poids brut, l'une des substances psychotropes contrôlées au niveau international les plus fabriquées.

Tableau 12. Méprobamate : fabrication et importations mondiales totales et nombre de pays importateurs (2023)

Substance	*S-DDD (en mg)*	*Quantité fabriquée (en kg)*	*Importations (en kg)*	*Nombre de pays importateurs*
Méprobamate	1 200	39 535,67	49 194,72	14

122. Bien que la fabrication et le commerce de méprobamate soient limités à un petit groupe de pays, le poids volumique élevé de cette substance nécessite, comme pour le GHB, la fabrication de quantités importantes pour que la demande puisse être satisfaite. Comme on le voit sur le tableau 12, 39,5 tonnes de méprobamate ont été fabriquées en 2023, ce qui représente une diminution sensible par rapport aux 97,1 tonnes déclarées en 2022. Comme les années précédentes, la Chine et l'Inde ont été les plus gros fabricants de cette substance en 2023, dont elles ont déclaré avoir fabriqué 26,0 tonnes et 13,5 tonnes, respectivement. Les stocks détenus par les fabricants de méprobamate au niveau mondial s'établissaient à 49,2 tonnes en 2023, c'est-à-dire nettement plus qu'en 2022 (37 tonnes). C'est la Chine qui en détenait les stocks les plus importants (40,6 tonnes), devant l'Afrique du Sud (3,8 tonnes). L'Inde et le Liban ont également détenu des stocks importants de cette substance en 2023, avec respectivement 1,9 tonne et 1,2 tonne.

123. Les importations totales de méprobamate ont augmenté de 4,4 tonnes entre 2022 et 2023, passant de 44,8 tonnes à 49,2 tonnes. L'Afrique du Sud a représenté à elle seule un peu plus de la moitié des importations totales de cette substance (26,4 tonnes), suivie par l'Inde (15,8 tonnes) et la République démocratique du

Congo (3,8 tonnes). Les exportations de méprobamate ont chuté entre 2022 et 2023, passant de 114,4 tonnes à 41,0 tonnes. La Chine et l'Inde, les principaux pays à fabriquer cette substance, sont aussi ceux qui en exportent le plus (21,7 tonnes et 17,7 tonnes, respectivement).

124. La fabrication et le commerce du méprobamate étant limités à un petit groupe de pays, la consommation en est également très limitée. En 2023, seuls 3 pays ont fourni des données sur leur consommation, contre 13 en 2022. Le niveau de consommation le plus élevé en 2023 a été signalé par le Liban, avec 0,21 S-DDD$_{ptpd}$, suivi par la Belgique (0,02 S-DDD$_{ptpd}$) et l'Inde (0,01 S-DDD$_{ptpd}$).

Buprénorphine

125. Des trois analgésiques inscrits au Tableau III de la Convention de 1971, seule la buprénorphine était présente en quantité non négligeable sur le marché licite en 2023. Opioïde utilisé principalement comme analgésique et dans le traitement de la dépendance aux opioïdes, elle a été importée par 97 pays et territoires cette année-là (voir tableau 13).

Tableau 13. Buprénorphine : fabrication et importations mondiales totales, et nombre de pays et territoires importateurs (2023)

Substance	*S-DDD (en mg)*	*Quantité fabriquée (en kg)*	*Importations (en kg)*	*Nombre de pays et territoires importateurs*
Buprénorphine	8	15 537,57	9 915,08	97

126. La fabrication mondiale de buprénorphine a amorcé une hausse progressive à la fin des années 90, époque à laquelle on a commencé à l'utiliser à plus fortes doses pour le traitement de la douleur et de la dépendance aux opioïdes. Après une baisse importante en 2010, la fabrication mondiale déclarée a augmenté régulièrement, atteignant 17,2 tonnes en 2018, puis elle est tombée à 10,5 tonnes en 2019, car aucune fabrication n'avait été signalée par le Royaume-Uni, qui en était le premier fabricant. En 2023, 15,5 tonnes au total ont été fabriquées, et quatre pays ont déclaré en avoir fabriqué des quantités importantes : le Royaume-Uni (5,9 tonnes), l'Allemagne (2,6 tonnes), les États-Unis (2,6 tonnes) et l'Inde (2,2 tonnes).

127. Le commerce de buprénorphine a diminué, passant de 13,5 tonnes importées en 2022 à 9,9 tonnes en 2023. Comme indiqué plus haut, le nombre de pays et territoires ayant déclaré des importations est resté stable, s'établissant à 97, et le principal importateur était les États-Unis (6,6 tonnes), suivi par la France (642,2 kg), l'Allemagne (484,4 kg), le Royaume-Uni (272,6 kg) et le Canada (246,9 kg). Trois autres pays en ont importé environ 100 kg chacun. En ce qui concerne les exportations, elles ont été principalement le fait du Royaume-Uni (5,3 tonnes), de l'Allemagne (1,6 tonne), et de la Tchéquie (1,3 tonne) en 2023.

128. En 2023, 64 pays et territoires ont communiqué des données sur la consommation de buprénorphine. La consommation de cette substance a été déclarée principalement en Europe et en Amérique du Nord, comme les années précédentes (voir tableau 14). La consommation la plus élevée pour 2023 a été déclarée par les États-Unis (8,84 S-DDD$_{ptpd}$), devant l'Islande (3,60 S-DDD$_{ptpd}$), le Royaume-Uni (2,45 S-DDD$_{ptpd}$), la Finlande (2,25 S-DDD$_{ptpd}$) et l'Australie et le Monténégro (chacun 2,11 S-DDD$_{ptpd}$). Cette dernière a fourni des données sur la consommation de la substance pour la première fois en 2023.

Tableau 14. Buprénorphine : consommation dans certains pays et territoires, classés par taux décroissants de consommation (2021-2023)

	S-DDD par millier d'habitants et par jour		
Pays ou territoire	*2021*	*2022*	*2023*
États-Unis	9,17	9,16	8,84
Islande	1,52	9,53	3,60
Royaume-Uni	3,30	2,13	2,45
Finlande	2,05	2,10	2,25

Français

Tableau 14. Buprénorphine : consommation dans certains pays et territoires, classés par taux décroissants de consommation (2021-2023) (*suite*)

	S-DDD par millier d'habitants et par jour		
Pays ou territoire	*2021*	*2022*	*2023*
Australie	–	–	2,11
Monténégro	2,21	2,10	2,11
Canada	1,92	2,01	2,10
Norvège	–	1,98	1,97
Portugal	0,47	1,48	1,69
Suède	1,55	1,59	1,64
France	–	–	1,48
Gibraltar	0,16	0,11	1,43
Autriche	1,26	1,25	1,22
Allemagne	1,26	1,66	1,01
Pologne	0,72	0,70	0,90

Préparations exemptées

129. Les obligations en matière de présentation de rapports prévues à l'article 16 de la Convention de 1971 exigent que les parties communiquent les quantités de substances psychotropes utilisées pour la fabrication d'autres substances psychotropes, de préparations exemptées et de substances non psychotropes. Ces utilisations de substances psychotropes se distinguent de la consommation déclarée de quantités utilisées à des fins médicales et scientifiques.

130. En vertu de l'article 3 de la Convention de 1971, les pays peuvent décider d'exempter de certaines mesures de contrôle des préparations contenant des substances psychotropes. Seules les préparations contenant des substances inscrites au Tableau II, III ou IV de la Convention peuvent être exemptées. Ces exemptions peuvent permettre à un pays de rendre certains médicaments plus facilement disponibles sur leur territoire ou de les échanger plus facilement.

131. En 2023, des quantités de 0,01 kg ou plus de cinq substances inscrites au Tableau II ont été utilisées pour la fabrication de préparations exemptées (voir tableau 15). Aucune utilisation de lévométhamphétamine n'a été signalée. Les années précédentes, les États-Unis avaient été le seul pays à avoir déclaré l'utilisation de lévométhamphétamine pour des préparations exemptées. L'Allemagne a été le seul pays à avoir déclaré l'utilisation de GHB pour des préparations exemptées, poursuivant la tendance observée depuis 2019. L'Azerbaïdjan a pour la première fois déclaré l'utilisation de métamfétamine pour fabriquer des préparations exemptées, et il a été le seul pays à le faire. En 2023, la Hongrie a déclaré avoir utilisé 1,38 tonne de racémate de métamphétamine. La quasi-totalité du *delta*-9-THC utilisé pour des préparations exemptées a été déclarée par l'Australie. En outre, les États-Unis ont utilisé moins de 0,01 kg de dexamfétamine pour des préparations exemptées.

Tableau 15. Substances inscrites au Tableau II utilisées pour la fabrication de préparations exemptées, par quantité utilisée (2021-2023)

	Quantité utilisée (en kg)		
Substance	*2021*	*2022*	*2023*
Racémate de méthamphétamine	0,03	127,49	1 388,89
Métamfétamine	0,05	0,01	412,00
Acide *gamma*-hydroxybutyrique	139,18	71,89	216,99
Delta-9-tétrahydrocannabinol	8,96	25,51	8,85
Dexamfétamine	0,01	0,05	0,01
Méthaqualone	<0,01	<0,01	<0,01
Méthylphénidate	<0,01	–	<0,01

Substance	Quantité utilisée (en kg)		
	2021	2022	2023
Phencyclidine (PCP)	<0,01	–	<0,01
Amfétamine	0,01	0,01	<0,01
Sécobarbital	0,02	<0,01	–
3,4-méthylènedioxypyrovalérone (MDPV)	0,00	–	–
N-benzylpipérazine	–	0,01	–
CUMYL-PEGACLONE	5,41	–	–
Éthylone	–	<0,01	–
Lévamfétamine	–	<0,01	–
Lévométhamphétamine	178,02	247,25	–

132. L'utilisation d'une quantité de 0,01 kg d'une substance inscrite au Tableau III pour la fabrication de préparations exemptées a été déclarée pour 2023 (voir tableau 16). Depuis 2017, les États-Unis sont le seul pays à déclarer l'utilisation de butalbital pour la fabrication de préparations exemptées. La majeure partie du butalbital qu'ils fabriquent sert à fabriquer ces préparations, notamment le phosphate de codéine et le paracétamol, ou d'autres substances non psychotropes. La quantité de buprénorphine utilisée dans des préparations exemptées diminue depuis 2020, seule une quantité négligeable en ayant été utilisée en 2022. En 2023, aucune utilisation de buprénorphine à cette fin n'a été signalée.

Tableau 16. Substances inscrites au Tableau III utilisées pour la fabrication de préparations exemptées, par quantité utilisée (2021-2023)

Substance	Quantité utilisée (en kg)		
	2021	2022	2023
Butalbital	7 584,69	5 303,81	978,69
Buprénorphine	1,45	0,01	–
Pentobarbital	<0,01	<0,01	<0,01
Amobarbital	<0,01	–	<0,01

133. L'utilisation d'une quantité de 0,01 kg ou plus de 17 substances inscrites au Tableau IV de la Convention de 1971 pour la fabrication de préparations exemptées a été déclarée par 12 pays pour 2023 (voir tableau 17). Dans l'ensemble, les tendances en matière de fabrication de préparations exemptées sont restées largement les mêmes que les années précédentes. La Fédération de Russie et l'Ukraine ont été les principaux utilisateurs de phénobarbital à cette fin. Toutefois, pour 2022, l'Algérie a déclaré pour la première fois en avoir utilisé plus d'une tonne. L'Allemagne a utilisé la majeure partie des benzodiazépines répertoriées dans le tableau 17 ainsi que du zolpidem et de l'oxazépam utilisés pour la fabrication de préparations exemptées.

Tableau 17. Substances inscrites au Tableau IV utilisées pour la fabrication de préparations exemptées, par quantité utilisée (2021-2023)

Substance	Quantité utilisée (en kg)		
	2021	2022	2023
Phénobarbital	17 956,20	18 049,26	61 380,65
Diazépam	2 408,39	1 597,26	1 918,90
Zolpidem	1 897,51	1 790,10	1 811,52
Oxazépam	2 377,52	1 405,61	1 680,15
Barbital	1 615,36	1 531,50	1 001,14
Témazépam	410,04	594,15	516,09
Bromazépam	609,38	513,54	515,04
Prazépam	312,00	211,88	311,80
Chlordiazépoxide	93,96	218,54	197,60

Français

Tableau 17. Substances inscrites au Tableau IV utilisées pour la fabrication de préparations exemptées, par quantité utilisée (2021-2023) (*suite*)

	Quantité utilisée (en kg)		
Substance	*2021*	*2022*	*2023*
Midazolam	277,62	228,28	183,37
Flurazépam	197,44	–	148,08
Lorazépam	224,94	85,69	94,44
Clonazépam	48,47	23,42	44,08
Alprazolam	32,69	43,47	33,72
Nitrazépam	59,03	18,00	26,00
Lormétazépam	37,66	3,63	11,43
Phentermine	8,21	0,01	0,01
Nordazépam	<0,01	<0,01	<0,01
Triazolam	–	–	<0,01
Flubromazolam	4,99	–	–

RÉGIME MONDIAL DES PRÉVISIONS RELATIVES AUX SUBSTANCES PSYCHOTROPES DESTINÉES À DES FINS MÉDICALES ET SCIENTIFIQUES ET TENDANCES RÉCENTES

Régime des prévisions relatives aux substances psychotropes et adhésion des pays

Introduction

134. Les personnes qui ont rédigé la Convention de 1971 n'avaient pas prévu, pour ces substances, de régime des prévisions semblable à celui qui avait été établi pour les stupéfiants placés sous contrôle en vertu de la Convention de 1961 telle que modifiée. Ce n'est qu'après l'entrée en vigueur de la Convention de 1971 que la communauté internationale a constaté qu'un régime mondial était nécessaire pour permettre aux pays d'indiquer leurs besoins annuels en substances psychotropes et de prévenir une production excédentaire ainsi que le détournement de ces substances du commerce international.

135. Dans ses résolutions 1981/7 et 1991/44, le Conseil économique et social a invité les pays à communiquer périodiquement à l'OICS des prévisions de leurs besoins médicaux et scientifiques annuels en substances inscrites aux Tableaux II, III et IV de la Convention de 1971. Les prévisions des besoins ne sont pas requises pour les substances inscrites au Tableau I. Depuis l'adoption de ces résolutions, l'OICS reçoit des prévisions de la part des pays et territoires et les met à la disposition de la communauté internationale de plusieurs manières différentes. Désormais, le régime des prévisions est un élément essentiel du contrôle du mouvement international des substances psychotropes.

136. Depuis que le régime des prévisions a été adopté, l'OICS conseille aux pays de lui communiquer au moins tous les trois ans des prévisions actualisées de leurs besoins licites annuels en substances psychotropes. Les pays sont également invités à communiquer toute modification de leurs prévisions relatives à telle ou telle substance, selon qu'il convient, par exemple si les besoins pour cette substance sont supérieurs aux prévisions établies précédemment.

Communication des prévisions et adhésion au régime des prévisions relatives aux substances psychotropes

137. En général, les pays et territoires adhèrent au régime des prévisions relatives aux substances psychotropes, bien que celui-ci ait été établi en dehors du champ d'application de la Convention de 1971 et qu'il soit entièrement facultatif. Tous les pays et territoires reconnus par l'Organisation des Nations Unies ont établi des prévisions pour au moins quelques substances placées sous contrôle en vertu de la Convention. Lorsqu'un pays n'a pas établi ses propres prévisions, ou n'est pas en mesure de le faire, l'OICS s'en charge afin que ce pays puisse importer les substances psychotropes les plus essentielles. Au cours des dernières années, le seul pays pour lequel l'OICS a dû établir des prévisions est le Soudan du Sud, en 2011.

138. Une fois établies, les prévisions relatives aux substances psychotropes restent valables, et les pays et territoires n'ont donc pas besoin de les actualiser chaque année, contrairement aux évaluations relatives aux stupéfiants placés sous contrôle en vertu de la Convention de 1961 telle que modifiée. Il est toutefois recommandé aux pays et territoires de mettre leurs prévisions à jour tous les trois ans afin qu'elles correspondent bien à leurs besoins à des fins médicales et scientifiques. Par conséquent, tous les pays et territoires ne soumettent pas de nouvelles prévisions chaque année, et s'ils estiment que leurs besoins sont satisfaits, ils peuvent ne pas modifier les prévisions établies.

139. Chaque année, de nombreux pays et territoires communiquent à l'OICS des prévisions actualisées relatives à certaines substances psychotropes. Chaque année de la période 2014-2023, 90 à 104 pays et territoires ont fourni un total de 2 690 à 3 700 prévisions relatives aux substances psychotropes (voir tableau 18). Chaque année de la même période, 88 à 104 pays et territoires ont soumis un total de 369 à 675 modifications de leurs prévisions établies pour les substances psychotropes. Au cours de cette période de 10 ans, 206 pays et territoires au total ont fourni au moins une prévision ou une modification d'une prévision établie pour une substance psychotrope.

Tableau 18. Prévisions relatives aux substances psychotropes et prévisions modifiées reçues des pays et territoires (2014-2023)

Année	*Prévisions*	*Pays et territoires ayant fourni des prévisions*	*Prévisions modifiées*	*Pays et territoires ayant fourni des prévisions modifiées*
2014	2 797	96	369	92
2015	2 690	92	513	98
2016	2 965	102	481	96
2017	3 192	104	398	88
2018	3 284	97	421	95
2019	3 700	97	500	90
2020	3 188	90	494	104
2021	2 983	94	607	90
2022	3 572	94	507	89
2023	3 680	94	675	94

140. Les substances pour lesquelles les pays et territoires ont fourni le plus de mises à jour ou de modifications des prévisions établies comptaient également parmi les substances le plus largement fabriquées et échangées. Au total, 146 substances, soit la quasi-totalité de celles inscrites aux Tableaux II, III et IV de la Convention de 1971, ont fait l'objet de prévisions ou de prévisions modifiées par au moins un pays ou territoire au cours de la période 2014-2023. Les substances qui ont fait l'objet du plus grand nombre de prévisions ou de prévisions modifiées en 2023 sont indiquées dans le tableau 19.

Tableau 19. Substances psychotropes ayant fait l'objet du plus grand nombre de prévisions ou de prévisions modifiées par les pays et territoires en 2023

Substance	*Prévisions*	*Substance*	*Prévisions modifiées*
Midazolam	100	Méthylphénidate	42
Diazépam	100	Phénobarbital	23
Phénobarbital	99	Dexamfétamine	20
Clonazépam	95	Pentobarbital	18
Alprazolam	93	Buprénorphine	17

141. Pour 2025, 70 pays et territoires ont fourni, au total, 2 428 prévisions relatives aux substances psychotropes. Pour les 144 pays et territoires qui n'ont pas fourni de prévisions actualisées pour 2025, celles qui avaient précédemment été établies pour 2024 seront reconduites. Contrairement au régime des évaluations relatives aux stupéfiants, les stocks et la consommation de substances psychotropes déclarés pour une année n'ont aucune incidence sur les prévisions relatives à ces mêmes substances pour l'année suivante. Les substances pour lesquelles le plus grand nombre de pays et territoires ont soumis des prévisions actualisées pour 2025 sont indiquées dans le tableau 20.

Tableau 20. Substances psychotropes ayant fait l'objet du plus grand nombre de prévisions par les pays et territoires pour 2025

Substance	*Prévisions*
Diazépam	70
Midazolam	70
Clonazépam	68
Phénobarbital	67
Alprazolam	65

142. Les prévisions établies pour 2025 pour tous les pays et territoires figurent dans les annexes publiées en ligne. Les pays et territoires pouvant mettre à jour à tout moment leurs prévisions relatives aux substances psychotropes, on trouvera les chiffres les plus récents sur le site Web de l'OICS.

Évolution des quantités de substances psychotropes évaluées par pays et territoires

143. Comme les pays et territoires ne sont pas tenus de mettre à jour leurs prévisions relatives aux substances psychotropes sur une base annuelle, les prévisions globales relatives aux substances psychotropes ne changent pas de manière significative d'une année à l'autre. Néanmoins, comme indiqué dans la section précédente, de nombreux pays modifient régulièrement leurs évaluations globales en cours d'année civile. L'analyse ci-dessous porte sur les évaluations telles qu'elles se présentaient à la fin de 2023 et 2024 et au début de 2025.

144. Pour 2025, les substances psychotropes ayant fait l'objet du plus grand nombre de prévisions en poids brut sont le phénobarbital (876,1 tonnes), le GHB (238,0 tonnes), le méprobamate (175,5 tonnes), le méthylphénidate (146,7 tonnes), le diazépam (124,1 tonnes), le pentobarbital (102,2 tonnes), le zolpidem (92,8 tonnes), la phentermine (62,2 tonnes), le chlordiazépoxide (57,8 tonnes) et le barbital (50,9 tonnes) (voir fig. 15). Les prévisions relatives au phénobarbital pour 2025 sont inférieures aux 923,8 tonnes prévues pour 2024. De même, les prévisions relatives au méprobamate, au diazépam et au barbital sont inférieures à celles des années précédentes. Les prévisions relatives au méthylphénidate ont augmenté d'environ 10 tonnes. En outre, les prévisions relatives à la phentermine pour 2025 ont presque doublé par rapport à celles de 2023, principalement en raison de l'augmentation des prévisions des États-Unis et du Mexique.

Figure 15. Substances psychotropes ayant fait l'objet du plus grand nombre de prévisions, en termes de poids brut (2023-2025)

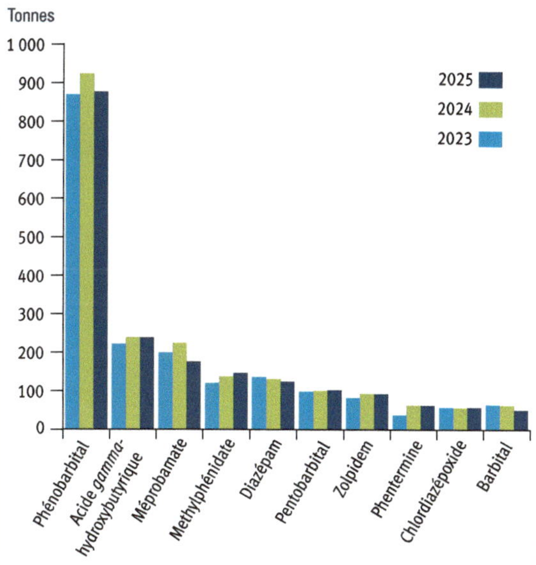

Figure 16. Substances psychotropes ayant fait l'objet du plus grand nombre de prévisions, en termes de S-DDD (2023-2025)

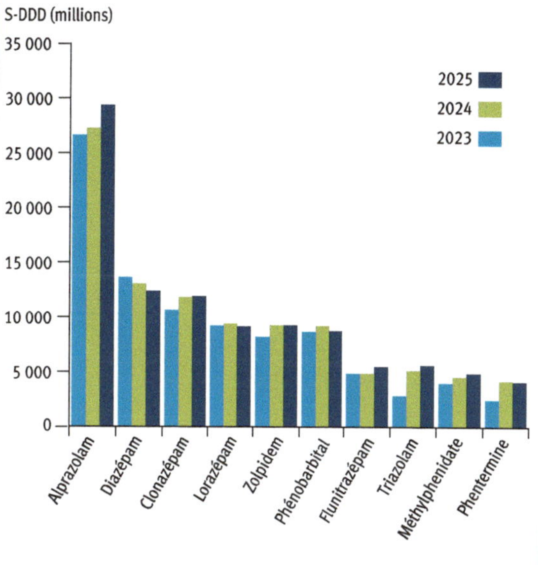

145. Considérées en termes de dosage (S-DDD), les substances psychotropes ayant fait l'objet du plus grand nombre de prévisions sont très différentes de celles exprimées en termes de poids brut. Pour 2025, les substances ayant fait l'objet du plus grand nombre de prévisions en termes de S-DDD sont l'alprazolam (29,4 milliards de S-DDD), le diazépam (12,4 milliards de S-DDD), le clonazépam (11,9 milliards de S-DDD), le lorazépam (9,2 milliards de S-DDD), le zolpidem (9,3 milliards de S-DDD), le phénobarbital (8,8 milliards de S-DDD), le flunitrazépam (5,5 milliards de S-DDD), le triazolam (5,6 milliards de S-DDD), le méthylphénidate (4,9 milliards de S-DDD) et la phentermine (4,1 milliards de S-DDD).

146. Comme on le voit sur la figure 16, sur le plan mondial, les prévisions relatives à l'alprazolam sont plus de deux fois supérieures aux prévisions relatives au diazépam, la deuxième substance ayant fait l'objet du plus grand nombre de prévisions. On remarquera que les prévisions relatives à l'alprazolam pour 2025 sont de 2,7 milliards de S-DDD supérieures à celles pour 2023. De même, les prévisions relatives au triazolam en 2025 ont doublé par rapport à 2023. En termes de poids brut et de S-DDD, les prévisions relatives au diazépam ont diminué. Les autres substances ayant fait l'objet du plus grand nombre de prévisions en termes de S-DDD n'ont connu que de légères modifications et fluctuations entre 2023 et 2025.

COMENTARIOS SOBRE LAS ESTADÍSTICAS COMUNICADAS RELATIVAS A LAS SUSTANCIAS SICOTRÓPICAS Y LAS PREVISIONES AL RESPECTO

Sinopsis

El análisis que figura en esta parte de la publicación técnica sobre sustancias sicotrópicas se basa en datos estadísticos y de evaluación presentados por los Gobiernos. La calidad de los resultados del análisis depende de la de los datos aportados.

En la primera sección del análisis se presentan las principales tendencias encontradas en los datos comunicados por los países y territorios, partiendo de un panorama general de la situación observada en 2023 con respecto a las 170 sustancias sicotrópicas sometidas a fiscalización internacional, y se destacan las principales tendencias que ponen de manifiesto los datos. También se proporciona información actualizada sobre la situación relativa a la fiscalización de las sustancias sicotrópicas y las modificaciones introducidas en las listas del Convenio sobre Sustancias Sicotrópicas de 1971.

La primera sección sigue con un análisis exhaustivo de las sustancias que suscitaron un mayor interés en 2023. El análisis se presenta desglosado por clase de sustancias, comenzando por el tetrahidrocannabinol (THC) y el *delta*-9-THC, los alucinógenos, la 3,4-metilendioximetanfetamina (MDMA), la psilocibina y la psilocina (psilotsina), seguidas de los estimulantes, las benzodiazepinas, los barbitúricos y otros sedantes hipnóticos, los ansiolíticos (concretamente el meprobamato) y la buprenorfina. Se examinan los datos más pertinentes sobre fabricación, importación, exportación, existencias y consumo notificado, y se comparan las tendencias derivadas de los datos correspondientes a 2023 con las de años anteriores. Se facilitan análisis e información adicionales sobre las sustancias utilizadas para la fabricación de preparados exentos.

La segunda sección ofrece un análisis del sistema de previsiones de las necesidades de sustancias sicotrópicas, incluido un examen de las previsiones anuales proporcionadas por los países y territorios.

Todos los datos utilizados respecto del consumo han sido proporcionados por los países y territorios como parte de los informes estadísticos que transmiten cada año a la Junta Internacional de Fiscalización de Estupefacientes (JIFE). A menos que se indique otra cosa, todas las cifras de consumo se expresan en dosis diarias definidas con fines estadísticos (S-DDD) por cada 1.000 habitantes por día, con la abreviatura S-DDD$_{pmpd}$. Esta unidad de medida fue adoptada por la Junta para medir el consumo de sustancias sicotrópicas de acuerdo con el enfoque utilizado por el Centro Colaborador de la Organización Mundial de la Salud en Metodología Estadística de los Medicamentos.

El análisis que figura en la presente publicación refleja únicamente los aspectos más destacados de la actividad lícita relacionada con las sustancias sicotrópicas sometidas a fiscalización internacional. Los datos completos para 2023, incluidos los datos sobre el consumo, y las previsiones para 2025 pueden consultarse en formato electrónico en el sitio web de la JIFE.

TENDENCIAS DE LOS DATOS COMUNICADOS SOBRE SUSTANCIAS SICOTRÓPICAS

Situación relativa a las sustancias sicotrópicas en 2023

1. Como se puede observar en el cuadro II de la presente publicación, al 1 de noviembre de 2024 163 países y 14 territorios habían presentado sus informes estadísticos anuales de conformidad con el artículo 16 del Convenio sobre Sustancias Sicotrópicas de 1971. Esas cifras reflejaban un aumento con respecto al año anterior, en que 155 países y 14 territorios habían presentado sus informes estadísticos anuales al 1 de noviembre.

2. La tasa de presentación de informes mejoró en todas las regiones en 2023 en comparación con 2022. Para 2023, al menos el 68 % de los países y territorios de cada región presentaron el informe estadístico anual requerido (véase el cuadro 1).

Cuadro 1. Estadísticas anuales sobre la presentación de informes por los países y territorios, por región, 2022 y 2023

	Número de países y territorios	
Región	*2022*	*2023*
África	39 de 57 (68 %)	42 de 57 (74 %)
América	36 de 45 (80 %)	37 de 45 (82 %)
Asia	40 de 48 (83 %)	41 de 48 (85 %)
Europa	41 de 43 (95 %)	42 de 43 (98 %)
Oceanía	13 de 22 (59 %)	15 de 22 (68 %)

3. A finales de 2023, el número de sustancias sicotrópicas que se habían sometido a fiscalización internacional ascendía a 170, frente a 167 a finales de 2022. En marzo de 2023, la Comisión de Estupefacientes decidió incluir la ADB-BUTINACA, la *alfa*-PiHP y la 3-metilmetcatinona en la Lista II del Convenio de 1971 y esas sustancias pasaron a estar sujetas a fiscalización internacional en noviembre de 2023.

4. Las sustancias sicotrópicas sometidas a fiscalización internacional comprenden varias categorías y tipos de drogas y se utilizan para tratar un gran número de problemas de salud. La mayoría de las sustancias sicotrópicas fabricadas y consumidas son sedantes hipnóticos, ansiolíticos y antiepilépticos, incluidos los barbitúricos y las benzodiazepinas. El otro grupo importante fabricado comprende los estimulantes, principalmente las anfetaminas y el metilfenidato. El resto de las sustancias que se fabrican habitualmente (alucinógenos, analgésicos y antianémicos) representan solo una pequeña proporción de la fabricación total de sustancias sicotrópicas.

5. Las tendencias generales de la fabricación de sustancias sicotrópicas sujetas a fiscalización internacional se mantuvieron en gran medida constantes en 2023 en comparación con 2022. En términos de peso bruto, la sustancia más fabricada a escala mundial fue el fenobarbital, con 374 t, una cantidad muy superior a la de cualquier otra sustancia (véase la figura 1). El metilfenidato fue la segunda sustancia más fabricada en todo el mundo, con 82,6 t, lo que, según datos de la Junta Internacional de Fiscalización de Estupefacientes (JIFE), supuso la mayor cantidad de esta sustancia jamás fabricada a nivel mundial en un solo año. La fabricación de meprobamato había ocupado el segundo lugar en 2022, pero disminuyó significativamente en 2023, ya que la fabricación notificada se redujo en más de la mitad, a 39,5 t.

6. Si se consideran en términos de dosis (S-DDD), las sustancias sicotrópicas fabricadas en mayores cantidades en 2023 presentan un panorama diferente en comparación con la clasificación por peso bruto (véase la figura 2). En 2023, el alprazolam fue la sustancia más fabricada, con más de 15.500 millones de S-DDD, casi el triple de los 5.800 millones de S-DDD notificados para el diazepam, que fue la segunda sustancia más fabricada. Las otras sustancias sicotrópicas fabricadas en mayores cantidades en 2023 en términos de dosis fueron el clonazepam (4.480 millones de S-DDD), el lorazepam (4.080 millones de S-DDD), el zolpidem

Figura 1. Sustancias sicotrópicas más fabricadas en el mundo, en peso bruto, 2023

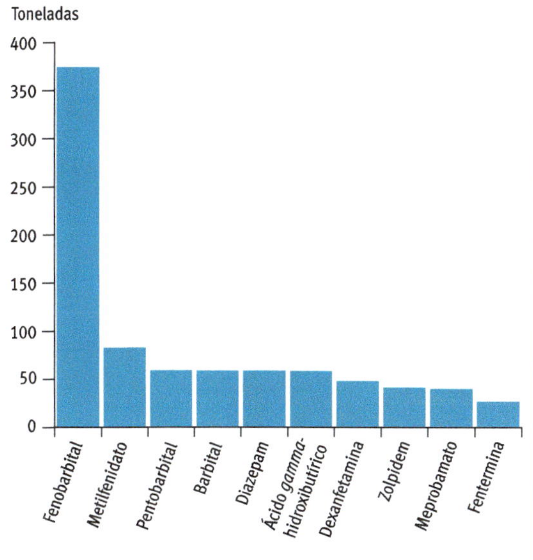

Figura 2. Sustancias sicotrópicas más fabricadas en el mundo, en S-DDD totales, 2023

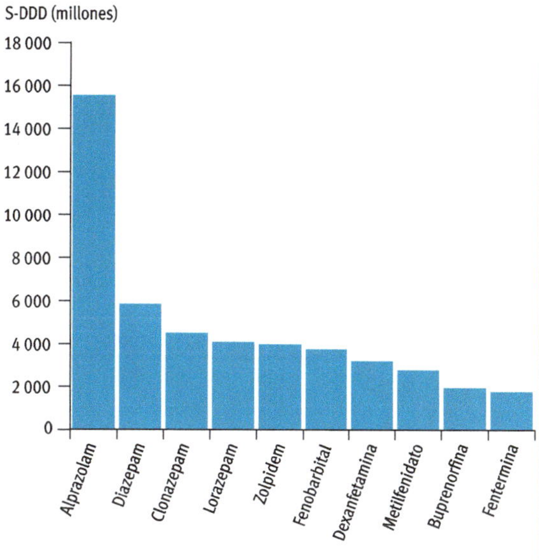

Español

(3.970 millones de S-DDD), el fenobarbital (3.740 millones de S-DDD), la dexanfetamina (3.180 millones de S-DDD), el metilfenidato (2.750 millones de S-DDD), la buprenorfina (1.940 millones de S-DDD) y la fentermina (1.770 millones de S-DDD). En 2023 se fabricaron otras 23 sustancias sicotrópicas en cantidades superiores a 100 millones de dosis.

7. En general, los principales países fabricantes de sustancias sicotrópicas siguen siendo los mismos que en años anteriores. En términos de peso bruto, la India fue el mayor fabricante en 2023, ya que es un fabricante importante de varios barbitúricos y benzodiazepinas. China fue el segundo mayor fabricante, debido sobre todo a su papel como gran productor de varios barbitúricos. Los Estados Unidos de América, Italia y Alemania completan los cinco mayores fabricantes por peso bruto. En términos de S-DDD, los cinco primeros países eran los mismos, pero con Italia en segundo lugar y China en cuarto. Cabe señalar que Suiza, que históricamente ha notificado cantidades mucho mayores de fabricación de sustancias sicotrópicas (más de 80 t en 2018), ha comunicado cifras muchas menores en los últimos años (7,4 t en 2023), debido sobre todo a que el país ha dejado de fabricar ácido *gamma*-hidroxibutírico (GHB) y *N*-bencilpiperazina (BZP).

8. En lo que al comercio internacional se refiere, seis benzodiazepinas se encontraban entre las sustancias sicotrópicas con que más se comerció en 2023 (véase el cuadro 2). El fenobarbital y el metilfenidato fueron, respectivamente, el barbitúrico y el estimulante sometidos a fiscalización internacional cuyo comercio estuvo más extendido. El zolpidem fue el sedante no benzodiazepínico no barbitúrico con que más se comerció. El número de países y territorios que notificaron importaciones de buprenorfina siguió aumentando en comparación con años anteriores, aunque el volumen de comercio de la sustancia fue más bajo en 2023 que en 2022.

9. Como en años anteriores, el diazepam fue la sustancia sicotrópica sometida a fiscalización internacional más importada en 2023, año en que 164 países y territorios notificaron importaciones de la sustancia por un total de 37,2 t, la cantidad más baja desde 2017. Del mismo modo, las importaciones totales de midazolam, fenobarbital y clonazepam en 2023 fueron entre un 10 % y un 30 % inferiores a las de 2022. Las importaciones de alprazolam aumentaron casi un 50 % en 2023 en comparación con 2022. Las demás sustancias más comercializadas no experimentaron cambios significativos en los volúmenes importados en 2023 en comparación con 2022.

Figura 3. Sustancias sicotrópicas más consumidas en el mundo, en S-DDD totales, 2023

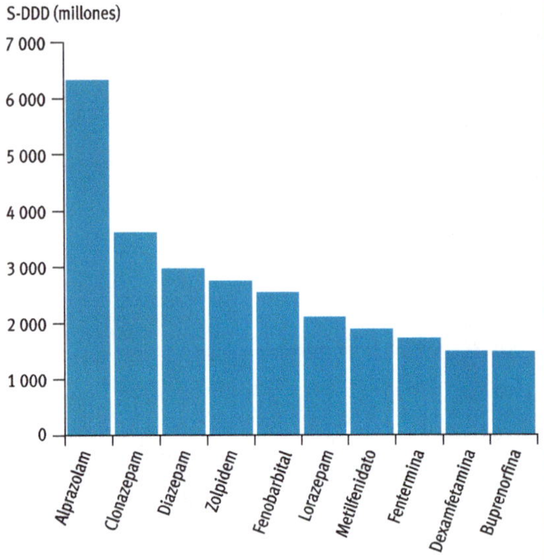

Figura 4. *delta*-9-Tetrahidrocannabinol: fabricación y existencias, 2014–2023

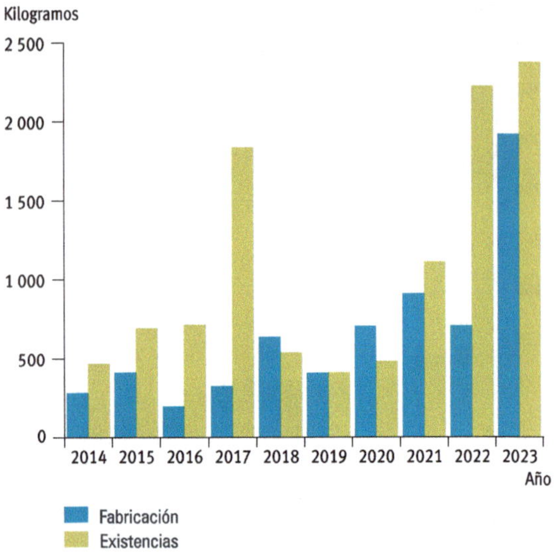

Cuadro 2. Sustancias sicotrópicas sometidas a fiscalización internacional cuyo comercio está más extendido, 2023

Sustancia	*S-DDD (mg)*	*Importación total (kg)*	*Importación total (millones de S-DDD)*	*Número de países y territorios importadores*
Diazepam	10	37 180,25	3 718,02	164
Midazolam	15	8 551,21	570,08	159
Fenobarbital	100	208 219,59	2 082,20	158
Clonazepam	4	11 374,47	2 843,62	142
Alprazolam	1	14 904,43	14 904,43	139
Lorazepam	2,5	8 540,29	3 416,12	126
Metilfenidato	30	59 952,31	1 998,41	120
Zolpidem	10	35 814,82	3 581,48	118
Bromazepam	10	15 861,96	1 586,20	113
Buprenorfina	8	9 915,08	1 239,39	97

10. Un total de 111 países y territorios (el 63 % de los que presentaron estadísticas anuales) proporcionaron datos sobre el consumo de al menos una sustancia sicotrópica en 2023, lo que representa un aumento con respecto a los 100 países y territorios que habían proporcionado esos datos en 2022. A nivel regional, las tasas de presentación de informes variaban considerablemente: en 2023 proporcionaron datos sobre el consumo 20 países y territorios de África (35 % del total de países y territorios de la región), 25 de las Américas (56 %), 22 de Asia (46 %), 35 de Europa (81 %), y 9 de Oceanía (41 %).

11. Dado que los valores de S-DDD establecidos para las sustancias sicotrópicas pueden variar enormemente entre las distintas sustancias (véase el cuadro III de la presente publicación), un análisis de los datos de consumo por peso bruto no reflejaría con exactitud las tendencias de consumo a nivel mundial. Los datos de consumo expresados en S-DDD totales reflejan mejor los hábitos de consumo de los países y territorios que comunican información y se prestan mejor al análisis. La figura 3 presenta las sustancias sicotrópicas más consumidas en el mundo en 2023 en términos de dosis totales (S-DDD).

12. En 2023, el alprazolam fue la sustancia más consumida, con más de 6.300 millones de S-DDD en todo el mundo, casi 1.500 millones más que en 2022. El consumo de clonazepam se duplicó con creces, de 1.600 millones de S-DDD en 2022 a 3.600 millones de S-DDD en 2023. El consumo de diazepam también aumentó, en

aproximadamente 1.000 millones de S-DDD hasta alcanzar casi 3.000 millones de S-DDD en 2023. Todas las demás sustancias más consumidas en 2023 experimentaron aumentos de consumo que de entre el 5 % y el 50 %. En cambio, el consumo mundial de estazolam se redujo drásticamente, de más de 3.100 millones de S-DDD en 2022 a 1.200 millones de S-DDD en 2023.

Tetrahidrocannabinol y *delta*-9-tetrahidrocannabinol

13. El tetrahidrocannabinol (THC) es un cannabinoide que se encuentra de forma natural en la planta de cannabis, pero que también puede obtenerse mediante procesos químicos. Todos los isómeros del THC están incluidos en la Lista I del Convenio de 1971, excepto el isómero *delta*-9-tetrahidrocannabinol (*delta*-9-THC), que está incluido en la Lista II. El uso lícito de THC y *delta*-9-THC ha sido limitado desde que estas sustancias se sometieron a fiscalización internacional; sin embargo, la actividad lícita relacionada con ellas ha ido en aumento en los últimos años, con el incremento del número de países que han autorizado el uso médico de algunos preparados de *delta*-9-THC.

Cuadro 3. Tetrahidrocannabinol y *delta*-9-tetrahidrocannabinol: fabricación lícita mundial total y existencias, 2023

Sustancia	*Fabricación (kg)*	*Existencias (kg)*
Tetrahidrocannabinol (todos los isómeros incluidos en la Lista I)	66,24	31,00
delta-9-Tetrahidrocannabinol	1 919,36	2 378,48

14. Como se muestra en el cuadro 3, la fabricación de THC sigue siendo muy limitada. Al igual que en 2022, Australia (62,93 kg) representó la mayor parte de la fabricación comunicada de la sustancia en 2023. El comercio de THC también es muy limitado y solo unos pocos países notifican importaciones o exportaciones. El Canadá fue el mayor exportador en 2023, con 560,81 kg, mientras que los Estados Unidos fueron el mayor importador, con 84,01 kg. La actividad de estos dos países representó casi todo el comercio en 2023 y solo unos pocos más declararon haber importado o exportado cantidades pequeñas. Australia fue el mayor consumidor de THC en 2023, con 46,99 kg de consumo declarado. Ningún otro país que proporcionó datos de consumo de THC informó del consumo de más de unos pocos gramos[1].

RECUADRO 1. TETRAHIDROCANNABINOL Y *DELTA*-9-TETRAHIDROCANNABINOL: CAMBIOS EN LOS INFORMES EN 2024

A partir de 2024, la Junta Internacional de Fiscalización de Estupefacientes aconsejó a los Gobiernos que revisaran sus procedimientos de presentación de informes con arreglo a la Convención Única de 1961 sobre Estupefacientes enmendada por el Protocolo de 1972 y el Convenio sobre Sustancias Sicotrópicas de 1971 en lo relativo al cannabis, así como a los cannabinoides derivados mediante procesos naturales y sintéticos.

La Junta recomendó que los países y territorios dejaran de comunicar las cantidades de extractos o tinturas de cannabis fabricadas, comercializadas, almacenadas, utilizadas o consumidas con arreglo a la Convención de 1961 en su forma enmendada. En cambio, los países y territorios deben informar de cualquier preparado o subproducto obtenido a partir del cannabis en términos de los cannabinoides, a saber, tetrahidrocannabinol (THC) y *delta*-9-THC, que contiene, que están sujetos a fiscalización en virtud del Convenio de 1971.

La Junta ha reconocido que la notificación sobre el THC y el *delta*-9-THC puede suponer un reto para algunos países y territorios en función de sus sistemas de fiscalización o recopilación de datos. La cantidad de isómeros de THC fabricados a partir de materiales naturales puede variar en función de la materia prima y del proceso utilizado para extraerlos.

[1] El consumo de tetrahidrocannabinol (THC) solo puede expresarse en términos de peso bruto, ya que no se ha establecido ningún valor para la dosis diaria definida con fines estadísticos (S-DDD) de la sustancia.

Español

15. Por lo que respecta al *delta*-9-THC, la actividad lícita relacionada con esta sustancia ha aumentado considerablemente en los últimos años, ya que cada vez más países han autorizado el uso de productos farmacéuticos y otros preparados que la contienen. La cantidad de *delta*-9-THC fabricado ha fluctuado desde 2014, pero ha ido en aumento en general desde 2020, cuando se notificó un total de 706,4 kg (véase la figura 4). En 2023 se fabricaron 1,92 t de *delta*-9-THC en todo el mundo; la mayor cantidad fue notificada por el Reino Unido de Gran Bretaña e Irlanda del Norte, con 602,8 kg, seguido de Sudáfrica (514,4 kg), Alemania (443,4 kg), Australia (207,2 kg) y los Estados Unidos (139,4 kg).

16. Las existencias de *delta*-9-THC de los fabricantes también han variado significativamente entre 2014 y 2023, pero han aumentado considerablemente desde 2020, cuando las existencias mundiales de los fabricantes se situaban en 481,9 kg. Esas existencias aumentaron a 1,11 t en 2021 y a 2,22 t en 2022. En 2023, las existencias de los fabricantes eran de 2,38 t a nivel mundial. El mayor poseedor de existencias en 2023 era el Reino Unido, con 1,1 t, seguido de Sudáfrica (426,5 kg), Alemania (398,4 kg), los Estados Unidos (313,1 kg) y Australia (98,3 kg). Otros 14 países comunicaron existencias de *delta*-9-THC, pero en cantidades muy pequeñas.

17. Se registra consumo de *delta*-9-THC en un número limitado de países; solo siete presentaron datos correspondientes a 2023. Antes de 2022, el consumo de *delta*-9-THC era relativamente bajo, y ningún país notificó un consumo superior a 0,3 $S\text{-}DDD_{pmpd}$. A partir de 2022, el consumo aumentó, sobre todo en Australia, que declaró 0,62 $S\text{-}DDD_{pmpd}$ ese año, mientras que otros países notificaron el consumo de menos de 0,3 $S\text{-}DDD_{pmpd}$. El consumo en 2023 aumentó considerablemente, ya que Sudáfrica comunicó por primera vez su consumo (5,53 $S\text{-}DDD_{pmpd}$), el más alto de todos los países que comunicaron datos de consumo, seguida de Australia (2,05 $S\text{-}DDD_{pmpd}$), Portugal (0,17 $S\text{-}DDD_{pmpd}$), Austria (0,06 $S\text{-}DDD_{pmpd}$), Suiza (0,05 $S\text{-}DDD_{pmpd}$) y el Reino Unido (0,05 $S\text{-}DDD_{pmpd}$).

Alucinógenos

MDMA

18. La MDMA es un estimulante con propiedades empatógenas, enactógenas y alucinógenas leves que está incluido en la Lista I del Convenio de 1971. Desde que la MDMA quedó sujeta a fiscalización internacional a mediados de los años ochenta, el uso lícito de la sustancia se ha limitado principalmente a la investigación científica y clínica. En los últimos años, unos pocos países han autorizado el uso de MDMA en casos excepcionales para determinados trastornos mentales relacionados con traumas, incluido el trastorno de estrés postraumático.

Figura 5. MDMA: fabricación, existencias y consumo, 2014–2023

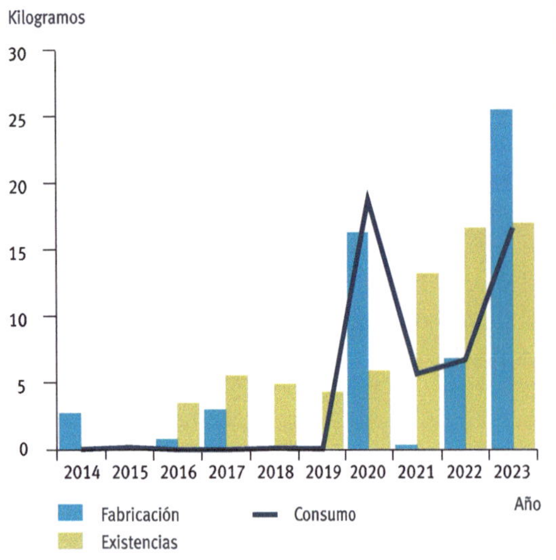

Figura 6. Fabricación de psilocibina y psilocina, 2014–2023

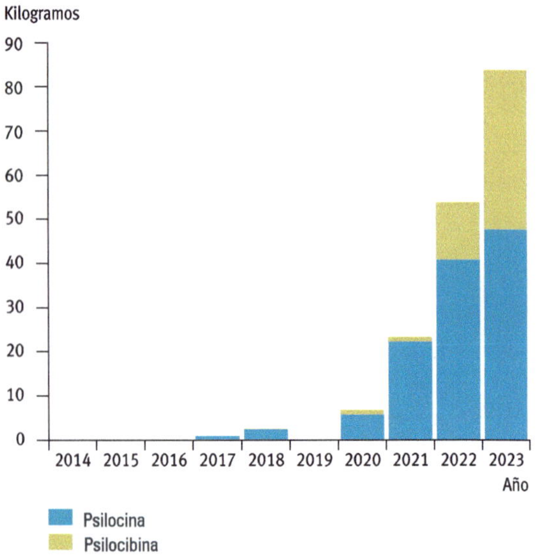

19. La actividad lícita relacionada con la MDMA fue escasa desde el momento en que la sustancia se sometió a fiscalización internacional hasta 2019, año en que aumentaron la fabricación y el consumo de la sustancia, probablemente como consecuencia de la creciente investigación sobre sus posibles aplicaciones terapéuticas. La MDMA solo se fabrica en unos pocos países, aunque el total de 25,54 kg comunicado para 2023 fue la mayor cantidad de esta sustancia fabricada en los últimos 10 años. El Reino Unido comunicó la fabricación de 22,34 kg de la sustancia, seguido del Canadá, con 2,68 kg. Australia, los Estados Unidos, el Reino de los Países Bajos y Suiza también comunicaron cantidades muy pequeñas. Desde que aumentó su fabricación de MDMA en 2020, el Reino Unido también ha sido el principal poseedor de existencias de la sustancia, con aproximadamente 12 kg en existencias cada año desde 2021. Las existencias mundiales de MDMA se situaron en 17,01 kg en 2023 (véase la figura 5).

20. Un total de 22 países y territorios comunicaron importaciones de MDMA en 2023, pero, como en años anteriores, las cantidades comercializadas fueron muy pequeñas. También fueron escasas las exportaciones de MDMA; el Canadá, el principal exportador, comunicó exportaciones de 0,67 kg en 2023. En general, el comercio de MDMA se ha mantenido prácticamente sin cambios durante los últimos diez años.

21. El consumo total de MDMA en 2023 ascendió a 16,67 kg; casi la totalidad de esta cantidad fue comunicada por el Reino Unido (15,87 kg)[2]. El Canadá, Suiza e Israel fueron los otros principales consumidores, con 0,24 kg, 0,21 kg y 0,18 kg, respectivamente.

Psilocibina y psilocina

22. La psilocibina y la psilocina (psilotsina) son sustancias alucinógenas incluidas en la Lista I del Convenio de 1971. Ambas sustancias se encuentran de forma natural en muchas especies de hongos de todo el mundo. La psilocibina es un profármaco que se convierte en psilocina en el cuerpo humano. Como en el caso de la MDMA, la actividad lícita relacionada con la psilocibina y la psilocina ha sido muy limitada desde que se sometieron a fiscalización internacional, pero dado que más países han autorizado la investigación y los ensayos clínicos con estas drogas, la fabricación, el comercio y el consumo lícitos de esas sustancias han aumentado en los últimos años.

23. Antes de 2020, la fabricación de psilocibina y psilocina era muy limitada, y la fabricación mundial total no superaba unas pocas docenas de gramos. En 2020, la fabricación mundial total de psilocibina aumentó a aproximadamente 1 kg y solo cambió ligeramente en 2021. En 2022, la fabricación mundial total aumentó a 13 kg, tras lo cual volvió a incrementarse, a 36,1 kg, en 2023 (véase la figura 6). En 2022 y 2023, el Reino Unido fue el principal fabricante de psilocibina, con 8,9 kg y 30,9 kg, respectivamente. El Canadá, los Estados Unidos y el Reino de los Países Bajos fueron los únicos otros países que comunicaron un nivel significativo de fabricación en 2022 y 2023.

24. Al igual que la fabricación, el comercio de psilocibina y psilocina estuvo muy limitado hasta 2020. Antes de 2020, las cantidades comerciales notificadas por los países y territorios rara vez superaban unos pocos gramos. En 2020, las importaciones mundiales totales de psilocibina y psilocina ascendieron a 0,46 kg y 0,04 kg, respectivamente. En cuanto a la psilocibina, la cifra aumentó a aproximadamente 1 kg en 2021 y se incrementó considerablemente en 2022, a 7,91 kg. En 2023, las importaciones mundiales de psilocibina se mantuvieron estables en 7,8 kg. Por lo que respecta a la psilocina, las importaciones mundiales totales ascendieron a 0,04 kg en 2020 y se han mantenido prácticamente sin cambios desde entonces. En 2023, las importaciones mundiales totales de la sustancia ascendieron a 0,06 kg.

25. Ningún país ni territorio ha notificado el consumo de psilocina en los últimos diez años. Históricamente, el consumo de psilocibina se ha limitado a no más de unas pocas docenas de gramos notificados por unos pocos países. En 2022, el consumo mundial aumentó significativamente, a 1,3 kg, principalmente como resultado del incremento del consumo en el Reino Unido (0,64 kg), Alemania (0,25 kg) y los Estados Unidos (0,25 kg)[3]. El consumo mundial total de psilocibina siguió aumentando hasta alcanzar los 3,86 kg en 2023, la mayor parte en

[2] El consumo de 3,4-metilendioximetanfetamina (MDMA) solo puede expresarse en términos de peso bruto, ya que no se ha establecido un valor de S-DDD para esta sustancia.

[3] El consumo de psilocibina solo puede expresarse en términos de peso bruto, ya que no se ha establecido un valor de S-DDD para esta sustancia.

el Reino Unido (3,1 kg), seguido de los Estados Unidos (0,46 kg) y Australia (0,13 kg). Otros seis países comunicaron consumo de la sustancia, pero en cantidades muy pequeñas.

Anfetaminas

26. En la Lista II del Convenio de 1971 figuran seis anfetaminas: los dos isómeros ópticos de la anfetamina (levanfetamina y dexanfetamina) y su mezcla racémica (anfetamina), así como los dos isómeros ópticos de la metanfetamina (levometanfetamina y metanfetamina) y su mezcla racémica (racemato de metanfetamina). Algunas de estas sustancias, en particular la dexanfetamina, suelen utilizarse para tratar a personas diagnosticadas de trastorno por déficit de atención con hiperactividad (TDAH).

27. En 2023, tres anfetaminas (anfetamina, dexanfetamina y metanfetamina) tuvieron una presencia destacada en el mercado lícito y 42 países y territorios importaron al menos una de ellas (véase el cuadro 4). De las tres sustancias, la que más se fabricó fue la dexanfetamina. La fabricación mundial de dexanfetamina aumentó en 2023 debido principalmente a un incremento de la fabricación comunicada por los Estados Unidos. La fabricación mundial de anfetamina se mantuvo prácticamente sin cambios de 2022 a 2023, y los Estados Unidos fueron el único fabricante. En cuanto a la metanfetamina, la cantidad fabricada volvió a los niveles de 2021, después de que en 2022 se hubiera comunicado un nivel muy bajo. El comercio de las tres sustancias aumentó entre 2022 y 2023, impulsado sobre todo por el incremento de las importaciones de anfetamina y dexanfetamina comunicado por Alemania.

Cuadro 4. Anfetaminas con una presencia destacada en el mercado lícito: fabricación e importación mundiales y número de países y territorios importadores, en orden descendente de la cantidad fabricada, 2023

Sustancia	*S-DDD (mg)*	*Fabricación (kg)*	*Importación (kg)*	*Número de países y territorios importadores*
Dexanfetamina	15	47 461,41	5 869,54	42
Anfetamina	15	16 766,23	835,63	31
Metanfetamina	15	596,89	1 200,37	24

Dexanfetamina

28. La fabricación total de dexanfetamina aumentó de 40 t en 2022 a 47,5 t en 2023 (véase la figura 7), ya que los Estados Unidos comunicaron un aumento de la fabricación de 10 t en comparación con el año anterior. Como viene ocurriendo desde hace muchos años, los Estados Unidos fueron el mayor fabricante de dexanfetamina

Figura 7. Dexanfetamina: fabricación, importación y existencias mundiales, 2014–2023

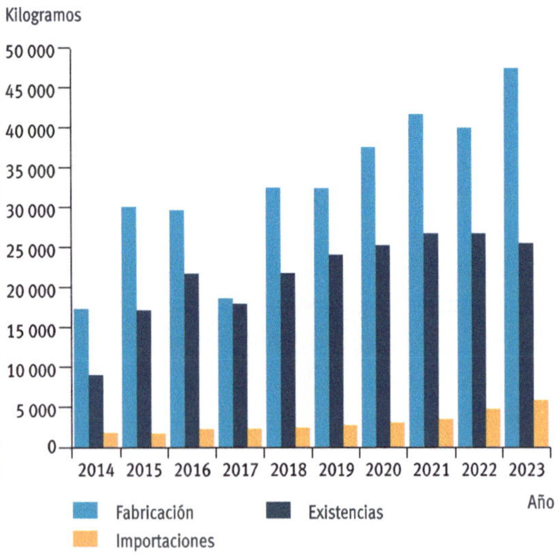

Figura 8. Dexanfetamina: cantidades utilizadas en la fabricación de sustancias no sicotrópicas, 2014–2023

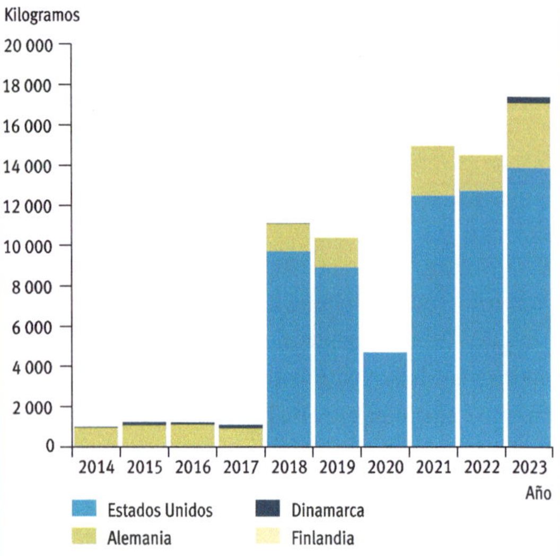

en 2023, con 42,6 t. Otros grandes fabricantes de la sustancia fueron Dinamarca (4,8 t) y Finlandia (84,1 kg). Francia, que históricamente ha sido un importante fabricante tanto de dexanfetamina como de anfetamina, se ha retirado del mercado y no ha informado de la fabricación de ningún tipo de anfetamina desde 2019.

29. Las importaciones mundiales de dexanfetamina han aumentado de manera constante durante los últimos diez años, de 1,79 t en 2014 a 5,69 t en 2023, año en que 41 países y territorios comunicaron importaciones. El mayor importador fue Alemania, que declaró 3,46 t, seguida de Australia (601,1 kg), el Canadá (505,9 kg), el Reino de los Países Bajos (265,1 kg) y Chile (237 kg); de este modo, los principales importadores de la sustancia no variaron respecto a 2022. Las exportaciones totales pasaron de 3,66 t en 2022 a 4,41 t en 2023, debido sobre todo al aumento de las exportaciones comunicadas por Dinamarca, que lideró las exportaciones en 2023, con 3,08 t, seguida de Francia (449,8 kg), los Estados Unidos (350,9 kg), Alemania (326,1 kg) y Croacia (108,4 kg).

30. En 2023, comunicaron consumo de dexanfetamina 27 países. El consumo global aumentó en la mayoría de los países que declararon consumo en comparación con el año anterior. Australia proporcionó datos sobre el consumo de la sustancia por primera vez en 2023. Los principales consumidores de dexanfetamina en 2023 fueron los Estados Unidos (11,50 $S\text{-}DDD_{pmpd}$), Australia (4,25 $S\text{-}DDD_{pmpd}$), Israel (2,57 $S\text{-}DDD_{pmpd}$) y el Canadá (2,04 $S\text{-}DDD_{pmpd}$). En todos los demás países que presentaron datos de consumo, las tasas comunicadas fueron inferiores a 2 $S\text{-}DDD_{pmpd}$. En el cuadro 5 se enumeran los diez países que comunicaron las mayores tasas de consumo de dexanfetamina en 2023.

Cuadro 5. Dexanfetamina: tasas de consumo en los diez países que comunicaron los mayores niveles de consumo en 2023, en comparación con 2021 y 2022

	S-DDD por 1.000 habitantes por día		
País	*2021*	*2022*	*2023*
Estados Unidos	8,57	8,05	11,50
Australia	—	—	4,25
Israel	1,52	2,07	2,57
Canadá	1,60	1,90	2,04
Chile	0,53	0,78	1,58
Islandia	0,91	0,94	1,27
Países Bajos (Reino de los)	1,10	1,26	1,26
Noruega	—	1,00	1,14
Suecia	0,92	0,89	0,92
Nueva Zelandia	0,58	0,07	0,58

31. En los Estados Unidos, la dexanfetamina se utiliza también para sintetizar lisdexanfetamina (*l*-lisina-*d*-anfetamina), profármaco de la dexanfetamina empleado en el tratamiento del TDAH que no está sujeto a fiscalización internacional. Los Estados Unidos comenzaron a notificar el uso de dexanfetamina para la fabricación de sustancias no sicotrópicas en 2018 y la cantidad utilizada ha seguido aumentando desde entonces. En 2023 se utilizaron 17,4 t de dexanfetamina para la fabricación de sustancias no sicotrópicas, la mayor parte por los Estados Unidos (13,9 t). Según la información facilitada a la Junta, toda esa cantidad se utilizó para la fabricación de lisdexanfetamina. Alemania y Dinamarca también comunicaron la utilización de dexanfetamina para la fabricación de sustancias no sicotrópicas en 2023, con 3,2 t y 302 kg, respectivamente (véase la figura 8).

RECUADRO 2. PROFÁRMACO DE LA DEXANFETAMINA: LISDEXANFETAMINA

Un profármaco es un compuesto inactivo que se activa una vez metabolizado en el organismo, liberando su componente activo para ejercer sus efectos. Un ejemplo es la lisdexanfetamina (*l*-lisina-*d*-anfetamina), un profármaco de la dexanfetamina, que es un estimulante del sistema nervioso central incluido en la Lista II del Convenio sobre Sustancias Sicotrópicas de 1971.

RECUADRO 2. PROFÁRMACO DE LA DEXANFETAMINA: LISDEXANFETAMINA *(continuación)*

La lisdexanfetamina fue sometida a un examen preliminar por el Comité de Expertos en Farmacodependencia de la Organización Mundial de la Salud en su 36ª reunión, celebrada en junio de 2014. En su informe, el Comité afirmó que se había establecido la seguridad y eficacia de la lisdexanfetamina en el tratamiento del trastorno por déficit de atención con hiperactividad (TDAH). Al mismo tiempo, el Comité llegó a la conclusión de que el hecho de que la lisdexanfetamina fuera un profármaco de la dexanfetamina implicaba la necesidad de una supervisión clínica y unas precauciones similares para el seguimiento y la fiscalización de este estimulante del sistema nervioso central. La sustancia nunca llegó al segundo paso del proceso de examen (examen crítico).

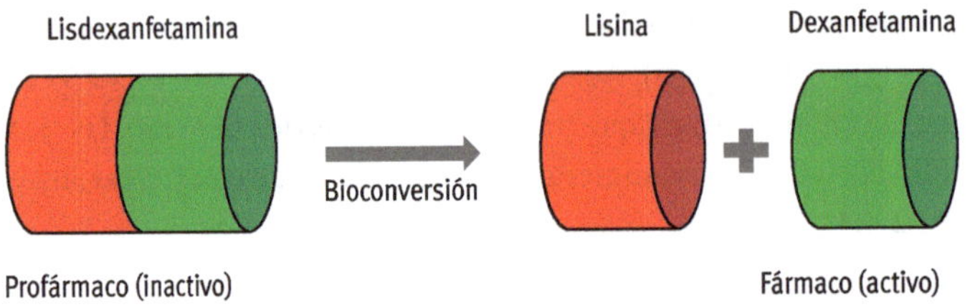

Utilizada principalmente en el tratamiento del TDAH, la lisdexanfetamina ha ganado protagonismo desde su comercialización en 2007 y se ha puesto en venta con los nombres de diversas marcas, como Vyvanse. Cuando se administra por vía oral y se metaboliza en el cuerpo humano, la sustancia se descompone en lisina, un aminoácido, y dexanfetamina. La lisdexanfetamina tiene un menor potencial de uso indebido en comparación con la dexanfetamina y actualmente no está sometida a fiscalización internacional; por consiguiente, las autoridades competentes no están obligadas a vigilar y comunicar datos estadísticos a la Junta Internacional de Fiscalización de Estupefacientes del mismo modo que en el caso de las sustancias sicotrópicas sometidas a fiscalización internacional. Sin embargo, algunos países sí han sometido la sustancia a fiscalización en el plano nacional.

Datos recientes muestran una tendencia al alza en la fabricación mundial de lisdexanfetamina, especialmente en los Estados Unidos, que representaron el 90 % de la fabricación mundial de dexanfetamina en 2023 y declararon que el 33 % de la sustancia se había utilizado para la fabricación de lisdexanfetamina. Algunos países europeos, como Dinamarca y Alemania, también han experimentado un repunte en el comercio de dexanfetamina. Alemania ha notificado un aumento del uso de la sustancia para la fabricación de sustancias sicotrópicas no sometidas a fiscalización. La Junta también ha observado un creciente interés de Bolivia (Estado Plurinacional de), Croacia y Panamá en la lisdexanfetamina.

Dado que en la actualidad la lisdexanfetamina no está sometida a fiscalización internacional, los datos de que dispone la Junta son facilitados por los países de forma voluntaria y, por tanto, no reflejan la situación mundial. No obstante, según los datos facilitados y las consultas recibidas por diversos países en relación con la lisdexanfetamina, parece que la sustancia está adquiriendo una presencia significativa en el mercado lícito internacional. Con el tiempo, el consumo de dexanfetamina con fines médicos puede verse desplazado por el de lisdexanfetamina.

La Junta agradece a los países que han transmitido voluntariamente información sobre la lisdexanfetamina y anima a todos los países y territorios a que en lo sucesivo comuniquen información sobre exportaciones e importaciones de la sustancia.

Anfetamina

32. La fabricación total de anfetamina aumentó ligeramente, de 16,1 t en 2022 a 16,8 t en 2023 (véase la figura 9). Como en años anteriores, los Estados Unidos fueron el principal fabricante de la sustancia, salvo algunos gramos fabricados por varios otros países. Las existencias mundiales de anfetamina cayeron de 22,5 t en 2022 a 19,6 t en 2023. La mayoría de esas existencias se encontraban en los Estados Unidos (19,2 t). El Canadá fue el otro gran

poseedor de existencias y comunicó 257,9 kg. Francia, que históricamente poseía grandes existencias de anfetamina, comunicó un total de 12,4 kg para 2023.

33. El comercio de anfetamina es relativamente limitado en comparación con las cantidades comercializadas de otras sustancias sicotrópicas. Desde 2018, las importaciones de anfetamina no han superado 1 t. En 2023, las importaciones mundiales de anfetamina se situaron en 835,6 kg, y casi la totalidad correspondió a Alemania (560,7 kg) y el Canadá (239,3 kg). Otros 29 países notificaron importaciones de la sustancia, pero solo en cantidades de unos pocos kilogramos o menos. Como principal fabricante de anfetamina, los Estados Unidos fueron el principal exportador de la sustancia y notificaron la exportación de 1,3 t en 2023, lo que representa un aumento con respecto a los 961,8 kg de 2022. Otros diez países notificaron exportaciones de anfetamina, pero solo en cantidades de unos pocos kilogramos o menos.

Figura 9. Anfetamina: fabricación, importación y existencias mundiales, 2014–2023

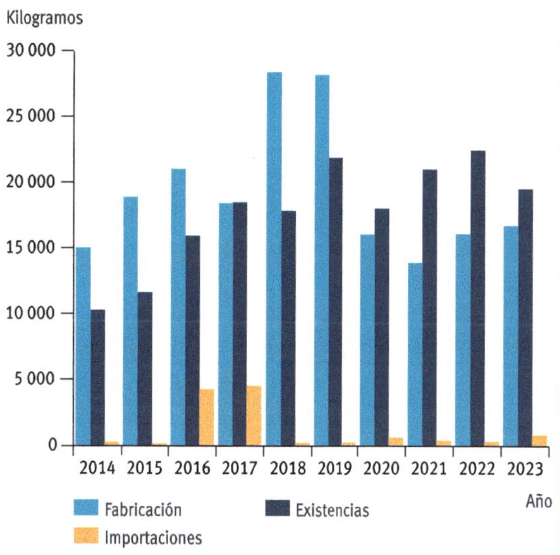

34. En total, 15 países o territorios informaron del consumo de anfetamina en 2023. El consumo global aumentó ligeramente, debido sobre todo a un incremento registrado en los Estados Unidos, pero muchos países y territorios comunicaron un consumo inferior al del año anterior. Los cinco principales países y territorios consumidores fueron los Estados Unidos (10,51 S-DDD$_{pmpd}$), el Canadá (0,98 S-DDD$_{pmpd}$), las Islas Turcas y Caicos (0,27 S-DDD$_{pmpd}$), Noruega (0,10 S-DDD$_{pmpd}$) y Suecia (0,09 S-DDD$_{pmpd}$).

Metanfetamina

35. La fabricación mundial de metanfetamina aumentó de unos pocos gramos notificados en 2022 a 596,8 kg en 2023. Hungría comunicó la fabricación de metanfetamina por primera vez desde 2020 y representó casi toda la fabricación de la sustancia en 2023. Otros dos países comunicaron la fabricación de unos pocos gramos de la sustancia. Las existencias mundiales de metanfetamina disminuyeron de 2,1 t en 2022 a 243,5 kg en 2023, ya que Francia no comunicó existencias de esta sustancia. Hungría acaparó casi todas las existencias mundiales.

36. Durante varios años, el comercio de metanfetamina fue mínimo, ya que solo se importaban o exportaban unos pocos gramos por año. En 2023, sin embargo, las importaciones y exportaciones mundiales aumentaron en 1,2 t cada una, debido a la exportación de esa cantidad de Francia a los Estados Unidos. El resto del comercio de metanfetamina siguió siendo limitado y otros pocos países comunicaron exportaciones e importaciones de apenas unos gramos.

37. Solo unos pocos países notifican el consumo de metanfetamina y en cantidades muy pequeñas. El único país que comunicó un consumo significativo en 2023 fue Macedonia del Norte (0,01 S-DDD$_{pmpd}$). Nueva Zelandia, que había notificado cierto consumo en años anteriores, no notificó ninguno en 2023.

Metilfenidato

38. Al igual que las anfetaminas, el metilfenidato es un estimulante incluido en la Lista II del Convenio de 1971 y también suele utilizarse para el tratamiento del TDAH. De los estimulantes incluidos en la Lista II, es el que más se fabrica y comercia, y 120 países y territorios comunicaron importaciones de la sustancia en 2023 (véase el cuadro 6).

Español

Cuadro 6. Metilfenidato: fabricación e importación mundiales y número de países y territorios importadores, 2022 y 2023

Año	S-DDD (mg)	Fabricación (kg)	Importación (kg)	Número de países y territorios importadores
2022	30	64 539,54	52 406,76	117
2023	30	82 645,73	59 952,31	120

39. La fabricación mundial de metilfenidato empezó a aumentar en 2012 y llegó a 74 t en 2016, el mayor nivel observado desde la década de 1990. En 2017, la fabricación mundial de la sustancia inició una tendencia descendente hasta situarse en 57,2 t en 2019. Posteriormente, la fabricación total se recuperó y alcanzó las 82,6 t en 2023, el nivel máximo registrado desde que la JIFE comenzó a recibir datos (véase la figura 10).

40. El aumento de la fabricación total de metilfenidato se debió principalmente a los incrementos comunicados por la India, Suiza y los Estados Unidos. En 2023, los Estados Unidos (58,4 t) volvieron a ser el principal fabricante. La India (11,2 t), Suiza (6,6 t), el Reino Unido (4,7 t) y España (1,1 t) también fabricaron cantidades considerables de la sustancia.

41. Las existencias mundiales de metilfenidato aumentaron casi 20 t, de 72,9 t en 2022 a 92 t en 2023. Ese aumento puede atribuirse sobre todo al Reino Unido, que incrementó sus existencias de 2,9 t a 17 t, y a Alemania, que pasó de 6,8 t a 8,9 t. Como en años anteriores, los Estados Unidos (44,5 t) representaron casi la mitad de las existencias mundiales en 2023. El Reino Unido (17 t), Alemania (8,9 t), Suiza (7,6 t) y el Canadá (4 t) fueron los otros grandes poseedores de existencias de metilfenidato.

42. El comercio internacional de metilfenidato siguió siendo muy activo en 2023: 120 países y territorios comunicaron importaciones de la sustancia y la cantidad de metilfenidato fabricada en los Estados Unidos que se exportaba a otros países fue en aumento.

43. El volumen de las importaciones de metilfenidato comunicadas por los países y territorios aumentó de 52,4 t en 2022 a 60,0 t en 2023. La mayor parte del aumento puede atribuirse a modestos incrementos de las importaciones de los principales importadores. Los cinco principales importadores de metilfenidato en 2023 fueron Alemania (10,5 t), el Canadá (6,3 t), Suiza (5,8 t), España (5,5 t) y Bélgica (3,5 t). Otros 13 países importaron más de 1 t de la sustancia. De los demás países y territorios que comunicaron importaciones de metilfenidato en 2023, 48 importaron más de 10 kg de la sustancia.

44. El volumen total de las exportaciones de metilfenidato comunicadas por los países y territorios aumentó de 49,8 t en 2022 a 60,9 t en 2023. Los Estados Unidos lideraron las exportaciones, con 17,4 t, frente a las 15,8 t de 2022. Entre los países exportadores también se destacaron Suiza (9,1 t), la India (8,7 t), el Reino Unido (6,1 t), Alemania (5,9 t) y España (5,1 t).

45. El uso de metilfenidato con fines médicos aumentó considerablemente en la década de 1990. La sustancia se utiliza para el tratamiento del TDAH, especialmente en los niños. También se receta para el tratamiento de la narcolepsia. El aumento de la fabricación y el uso de metilfenidato se deben principalmente a la evolución de la situación en los Estados Unidos, donde la sustancia se suele recetar para el tratamiento del TDAH y también es objeto de múltiples campañas publicitarias, también dirigidas directamente a posibles consumidores.

46. El número de países y territorios que proporcionaron datos sobre el consumo de metilfenidato aumentó de 66 en 2022 a 80 en 2023. La diferencia entre los índices de consumo más elevados y los más bajos siguió siendo considerable, principalmente debido a la importante cantidad notificada por Islandia, que ha mostrado niveles de consumo de metilfenidato sistemáticamente altos durante muchos años.

Figura 10. Metilfenidato: fabricación, importación y existencias mundiales, 2014–2023

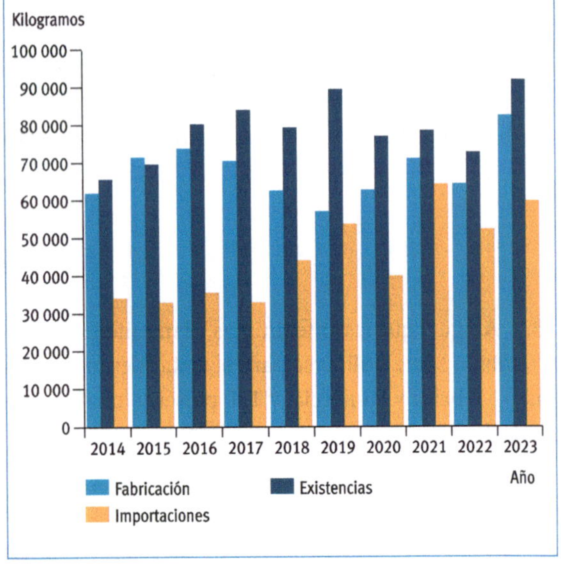

47. En comparación con las cifras comunicadas correspondientes a 2022, el consumo de metilfenidato en Islandia aumentó de 29,47 S-DDDpmpd a 34,50 S-DDDpmpd; el país notificó el mayor consumo mundial en 2023, como viene ocurriendo desde hace muchos años. El consumo de esta sustancia aumentó ligeramente en casi todos los países que facilitaron datos (véase el cuadro 7).

Cuadro 7. Metilfenidato: tasas de consumo en los diez países que comunicaron los mayores niveles de consumo en 2023, en comparación con 2021 y 2022

	S-DDD por 1.000 habitantes por día		
País	*2021*	*2022*	*2023*
Islandia	53,33	29,47	34,50
Dinamarca	9,39	10,63	12,88
Canadá	10,01	11,14	12,15
Nueva Zelandia	7,70	5,35	9,87
Suecia	8,57	9,01	9,61
Noruega	—	8,38	9,14
Países Bajos (Reino de los)	7,74	8,33	9,11
Israel	10,05	7,73	8,36
Estados Unidos	7,34	6,90	7,14
Australia	—	—	6,38

Español

Fentermina

48. De los estimulantes no incluidos en la Lista II del Convenio de 1971, solo uno, la fentermina, tuvo una presencia destacada en el mercado lícito en 2023. La fentermina ha seguido siendo sistemáticamente el estimulante no anfetamínico más fabricado y se utiliza en medicina como inhibidor del apetito para el control a corto plazo de la obesidad.

49. La fabricación mundial de fentermina siguió disminuyendo en 2023 debido principalmente a las reducciones comunicadas por Alemania. El volumen de importaciones de la sustancia aumentó en 2023 debido a un incremento significativo de las importaciones de los Estados Unidos. En total, 43 países y territorios comunicaron importaciones de fentermina en 2023 (véase el cuadro 8). Las tendencias de consumo se mantuvieron prácticamente sin cambios, y Nueva Zelandia y Chile fueron los mayores consumidores per cápita en 2023.

Cuadro 8. Fentermina: fabricación e importación mundiales, 2023

Sustancia	*S-DDD (mg)*	*Fabricación (kg)*	*Importación (kg)*	*Número de países y territorios importadores*
Fentermina	15	26 551,94	24 014,82	43

50. La fabricación mundial de fentermina cayó por segundo año consecutivo, de 29,1 t en 2022 a 26,6 t en 2023, debido a una reducción interanual de 9 t comunicada por los Estados Unidos, mientras que Alemania comunicó un aumento de 7 t. Alemania fue el mayor fabricante de fentermina en 2023, con 19,3 t, seguida de los Estados Unidos (3,7 t), Italia (2,38 t) y la India (675,1 kg). Las existencias mundiales de fentermina también cayeron por segundo año consecutivo, de 27,5 t en 2022 a 23,3 t en 2023. La mayor parte de las existencias correspondió a los Estados Unidos (13,9 t), seguidos de Alemania (4,6 t) e Italia (1 t). Otros 21 países comunicaron pequeñas existencias de la sustancia.

51. Las importaciones mundiales de fentermina aumentaron en 2023, cuando 43 países y territorios informaron de un total de 24 t importadas, lo que representa un incremento con respecto a las 19,4 t de 2022. Al igual que en 2022, los Estados Unidos (9,2 t) siguieron siendo el principal importador de la sustancia, seguidos de México (5 t), Chile (2,7 t) y la República de Corea (1,7 t). Las exportaciones mundiales de fentermina aumentaron a 24,6 t en 2023 y Alemania siguió siendo el principal exportador de la sustancia (17 t). Otros exportadores importantes fueron Italia (2,8 t), Australia (962,4 kg), la India (946,5 kg), Suiza (888,6 kg) y los Estados Unidos (887,5 kg).

52. Veinticinco países y territorios comunicaron datos sobre el consumo de fentermina en 2023; los que comunicaron mayor consumo fueron Nueva Zelandia (14,35 S-DDDpmpd), Chile (9,18 S-DDDpmpd), los Estados Unidos (8,56 S-DDDpmpd), México (8,31 S-DDDpmpd) y la República de Corea (7,95 S-DDDpmpd), los mismos cinco que el año anterior. Aunque los países con mayor consumo de fentermina se mantuvieron sin cambios respecto a 2022, el consumo global disminuyó en todos los países y territorios en 2023.

Benzodiazepinas

53. Las benzodiazepinas son una clase de sustancias de la Lista IV del Convenio de 1971 que se utilizan para el tratamiento de una serie de afecciones. Algunas de las benzodiazepinas que más se recetan se utilizan para tratar la ansiedad, los trastornos de pánico, la depresión y el insomnio; otras también se emplean como inductores de la anestesia general y la sedación antes de una intervención quirúrgica y para tratar los síntomas de la abstinencia alcohólica y la agitación asociada al consumo de drogas. El comercio de benzodiazepinas ha sido un fenómeno mundial durante décadas. Durante el período 2014–2023, prácticamente todos los países y territorios informaron a la JIFE de que habían comerciado con al menos una benzodiazepina en cantidades superiores a 1 kg.

54. A principios de la década de 1980, las benzodiazepinas empezaron a estar sujetas a fiscalización internacional. Con el tiempo, las medidas de fiscalización se han ampliado para incluir sustancias adicionales, y en la actualidad 41 benzodiazepinas están sujetas a fiscalización internacional, incluidas cuatro clasificadas como nuevas sustancias psicoactivas.

55. De las 41 benzodiazepinas sujetas a fiscalización internacional, 16 tuvieron una presencia destacada en el mercado lícito en 2023 (véase el cuadro 9). Como en años anteriores, las benzodiazepinas con las que más se comerció en 2023 fueron el diazepam, el midazolam, el clonazepam, el alprazolam y el lorazepam, y 126 o más países y territorios comunicaron que habían importado cada una de esas sustancias. En comparación con 2022, el número de países y territorios que comunicaron importaciones de esas benzodiazepinas solo cambió ligeramente.

Cuadro 9. Benzodiazepinas con una presencia destacada en el mercado lícito: fabricación mundial y número de países y territorios importadores, por fabricación en S-DDD, 2023

Sustancia	*S-DDD (mg)*	*Fabricación (kg)*	*Fabricación (millones de S-DDD)*	*Número de países y territorios importadores*
Alprazolam	1	15 550,22	15 550,22	139
Diazepam	10	58 226,30	5 822,63	164
Clonazepam	4	17 938,95	4 484,74	142
Lorazepam	2,5	10 198,60	4 079,44	126
Bromazepam	10	8 959,04	895,90	113
Clordiazepóxido	30	22 826,23	760,87	83
Midazolam	15	9 157,37	610,49	159
Nitrazepam	5	2 860,76	572,15	54
Flunitrazepam	1	543,73	543,73	31
Clobazam	20	8 734,77	436,74	95
Oxazepam	50	18 799,45	375,99	53
Temazepam	20	6 853,11	342,66	32
Triazolam	0,25	57,70	230,79	39
Prazepam	30	3 900,33	130,01	27
Flurazepam	30	2 757,74	91,92	21
Clorazepato	20	1 486,93	74,35	44

56. En 2023, la fabricación total comunicada de las benzodiazepinas que tenían una presencia destacada en el mercado lícito alcanzó aproximadamente 189 t, lo que supone un aumento en comparación con 2022. Si bien se comunicó fabricación de benzodiazepinas en muchas regiones del mundo, el 96 % del total fabricado estuvo concentrado en cuatro países: Italia (41 %), India (37 %), China (9 %) y Brasil (9 %). A pesar de una ligera reducción de la fabricación, Italia sigue siendo el principal fabricante. La fabricación en la India aumentó un 31 % respecto

Figura 11. Benzodiazepinas con una presencia destacada en el mercado lícito: porcentaje de la fabricación mundial por sustancia, basado en el peso bruto, 2023

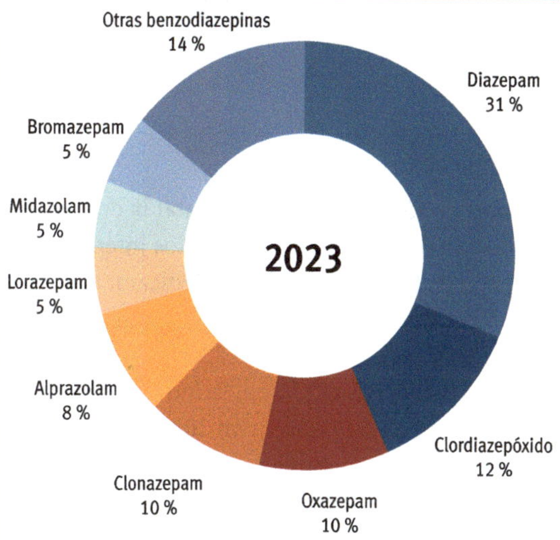

Figura 12. Diazepam: número de países y territorios que comunicaron consumo, por región, 2019–2023

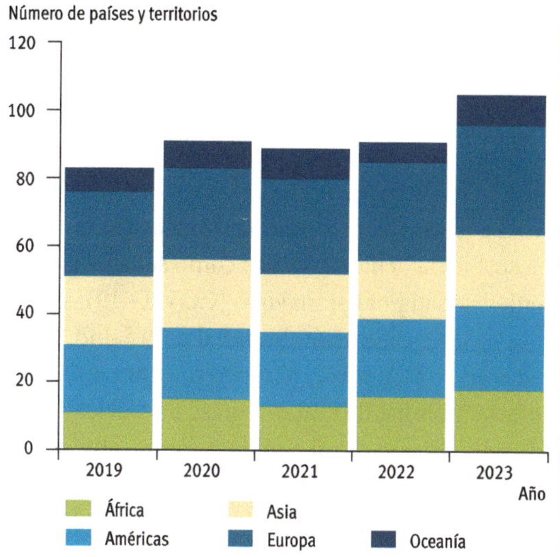

a 2022 y alcanzó un máximo histórico, mientras que China casi duplicó su fabricación de 2022 a 2023. En términos de peso bruto, ocho benzodiazepinas (diazepam, clordiazepóxido, oxazepam, clonazepam, alprazolam, lorazepam, midazolam y bromazepam) representaron el 86 % de la fabricación total en 2023 (véase la figura 11).

Diazepam

57. El diazepam fue la benzodiazepina más fabricada en 2023 en términos de peso bruto (58,2 t), y representó el 31 % de la fabricación total de las benzodiazepinas que tenían una presencia destacada en el mercado lícito. La fabricación mundial de diazepam ha fluctuado marcadamente en años recientes. La fabricación de esta sustancia en Italia alcanzó un máximo de 29,2 t en 2021, pero luego se redujo drásticamente, a 17,9 t en 2023. Por el contrario, la India aumentó sustancialmente su fabricación, de 12,7 t en 2022 a 20,9 t en 2023. La fabricación en China ha fluctuado, cayendo a 1,3 t en 2020 y recuperándose a 11,4 t en 2023. Tras un mínimo de 0,4 t en 2022, la fabricación en el Brasil volvió a aumentar, a 7,8 t, en 2023. A nivel mundial, más del 99 % de la fabricación de diazepam en 2023 correspondió a cuatro países: India, Italia, China y Brasil. Las existencias totales en manos de fabricantes de todos los países y territorios disminuyeron ligeramente, pasando de 42,9 t en 2022 a 40,3 t en 2023. Los países con las mayores existencias de diazepam en 2023 fueron China (10,4 t), Italia (8,3 t), el Brasil (6,2 t) y Dinamarca (3,7 t).

58. El diazepam fue también la sustancia sicotrópica sometida a fiscalización internacional con que más se comerció en 2023: 164 países y territorios comunicaron importaciones de la sustancia. Las importaciones mundiales de diazepam habían aumentado constantemente, de 32,5 t en 2017 a un máximo de 66,4 t en 2021. Sin embargo, las importaciones siguieron después una tendencia a la baja, y disminuyeron a 44,4 t en 2022 y a 37,2 t en 2023. El número de países y territorios que importan diazepam alcanzó un máximo de 176 en 2018 y luego fluctuó en los años siguientes. Como ya se ha indicado, 164 países y territorios notificaron importaciones de la sustancia en 2023, lo que supone un aumento con respecto a los 160 que lo habían hecho en 2022. Ghana, España, los Estados Unidos, la República Democrática del Congo, Chequia, Alemania, Francia, Bangladesh, el Japón y Serbia (en orden descendente de las cantidades importadas) comunicaron importaciones de más de 1 t en 2023, que en conjunto supusieron aproximadamente el 60 % del total de las importaciones mundiales. Los principales países exportadores en 2023 fueron Italia (16,3 t), la India (10,2 t), Dinamarca (2,7 t), Chequia (2,2 t), Alemania (1,8 t), China (1,7 t), Suiza (1,1 t) y España (0,7 t). En conjunto, esos países sumaron el 93 % del total de las exportaciones mundiales de la sustancia.

59. Entre los países y territorios que proporcionaron datos, el número que comunicó datos de consumo de diazepam aumentó significativamente, de 91 en 2022 a 105 en 2023 (véase la figura 12). Cabo Verde comunicó

el nivel más alto de consumo de diazepam en 2023, con 20,90 S-DDD_{pmpd}, un aumento significativo en comparación con las 5,74 S-DDD_{pmpd} de 2022. Montenegro (14,37 S-DDD_{pmpd}), Portugal (13,88 S-DDD_{pmpd}) y España (13,68 S-DDD_{pmpd}) estuvieron entre los otros países que comunicaron un consumo superior a 10 S-DDD_{pmpd} en 2023. El Brasil también experimentó un fuerte aumento del consumo, alcanzando 12,03 S-DDD_{pmpd} en 2023, frente a 1,41 S-DDD_{pmpd} de 2022. Bosnia y Herzegovina informó de un nivel de consumo de 10,71 S-DDD_{pmpd} en 2023, mientras que Guyana informó de 9,30 S-DDD_{pmpd}.

Midazolam

60. La fabricación de midazolam alcanzó un nivel sin precedentes de 25 t en 2021, al aumentar la demanda de esta sustancia debido a su uso como sedante para pacientes ingresados en unidades de cuidados intensivos con la enfermedad por coronavirus (COVID-19), así como a su inclusión en la Lista Modelo de Medicamentos Esenciales de la Organización Mundial de la Salud. La fabricación cayó bruscamente en 2022, a 13,5 t, y nuevamente, a 9,2 t, en 2023, pero se mantuvo muy por encima de los niveles anteriores a 2021. Desde 2016, más del 98 % de la oferta mundial de midazolam se ha fabricado en cinco países, a saber, el Brasil, China, la India, Israel e Italia. El Brasil informó de un aumento significativo en su fabricación, de 1,4 t en 2022 a 3,1 t en 2023. La fabricación en la India siguió disminuyendo y cayó de 4,4 t en 2022 a 2,9 t en 2023. Italia también registró una disminución de la fabricación, de 4,4 t en 2022 a 2,3 t en 2023. Israel, uno de los principales fabricantes en años anteriores, no comunicó fabricación en 2023. China fabricó 0,8 t, lo que supone un aumento respecto a las 0,7 t de 2022. Las existencias mundiales de midazolam que estaban en posesión de los fabricantes llegaron a 8,4 t en 2023, lo que supuso una disminución respecto de las 14,4 t registradas en 2022. Las mayores existencias estaban en poder del Brasil (1,8 t), Italia (1,1 t), Francia (1,0 t), la India (0,9 t) y los Estados Unidos (0,9 t). La disminución de las existencias de midazolam en manos de los fabricantes a nivel mundial de 14,4 t en 2022 a 8,4 t en 2023 se atribuye principalmente a las reducciones significativas de los niveles de existencias en el Brasil (de 4,5 t a 1,8 t) y la India (de 1,4 t a 0,9 t), entre otros países.

61. De 2014 a 2023 se comunicó un volumen total de importaciones de midazolam de 10,7 t en promedio por año a nivel mundial. Si bien el número de países y territorios que notificaron importaciones se ha mantenido relativamente estable, el volumen ha aumentado considerablemente, y en 2021 alcanzó el máximo nivel en diez años, 18,2 t, impulsado por la demanda relacionada con la pandemia de COVID-19. En 2022, las importaciones disminuyeron a 12,6 t, seguidas de un nuevo descenso a 8,6 t notificado por un total de 159 países y territorios en 2023. El mayor importador de midazolam en 2023 fue Alemania (2,9 t); los demás países y territorios comunicaron cantidades de importación significativamente inferiores. La disminución general de las importaciones se debió principalmente a las grandes reducciones de los principales importadores de años anteriores, como el Brasil, que importó solo 0,2 t frente a las 2,5 t de 2022, y Türkiye, que comunicó un drástico descenso de 1,2 t en 2022 a solo 80 kg en 2023. De modo similar, las exportaciones mundiales de midazolam disminuyeron de 20,9 t en 2021 a 12,6 t en 2022 y luego a 9,1 t en 2023. Las exportaciones estuvieron encabezadas por Italia (3,5 t), Alemania (2 t) y la India (1,2 t), mientras que otros exportadores clave experimentaron notables disminuciones. Por ejemplo, las exportaciones de Israel cayeron de 1,9 t en 2022 a solo 471 kg en 2023. Asimismo, las exportaciones de la India disminuyeron de 2,8 t en 2022 a 1,2 t en 2023.

62. Para 2023, facilitaron datos de consumo de midazolam 100 países y territorios. Grecia (4,01 S-DDD_{pmpd}), San Martín (3,97 S-DDD_{pmpd}), el Brasil (3,18 S-DDD_{pmpd}) y el Uruguay (2,30 S-DDD_{pmpd}) comunicaron las tasas más elevadas de consumo de midazolam. Sin embargo, muchos países y territorios registraron disminuciones significativas del consumo en comparación con años anteriores. Grecia, a pesar de encabezar la lista, registró una reducción desde las 7,08 S-DDD_{pmpd} en 2022. Del mismo modo, el consumo declarado por Türkiye, que había aumentado a 2,34 S-DDD_{pmpd} en 2022, disminuyó a solo 0,03 S-DDD_{pmpd} en 2023. Israel también experimentó una disminución, de 1,41 S-DDD_{pmpd} en 2022 a 0,29 S-DDD_{pmpd} en 2023.

Clonazepam

63. El clonazepam, la única benzodiazepina antiepiléptica sometida a fiscalización internacional, también se utiliza para el tratamiento del trastorno de pánico y la ansiedad. En 2023, la fabricación mundial de clonazepam alcanzó un máximo histórico. Tras aumentar a 17,2 t en 2021 y luego disminuir a 10,7 t en 2022, la fabricación

total subió a 17,9 t en 2023. La India fue el mayor fabricante, con 11,4 t en 2023, más del doble de las 5,2 t registradas en 2022. Le siguió el Brasil, con 3,6 t, frente a las 2,1 t de 2022. Otros fabricantes importantes fueron Italia (1,6 t) y China (1,04 t). Suiza, que había fabricado grandes cantidades de la sustancia en años anteriores, solo comunicó 3,7 kg en 2022 y no notificó fabricación alguna en 2023. Las existencias de clonazepam disminuyeron ligeramente, de 6,6 t en 2022 a 6,4 t en 2023. Las existencias en Suiza pasaron de 1 t en 2022 a 472 kg en 2023. México, que tenía 1 t de existencias en 2022, no comunicó existencias en 2023. Al mismo tiempo, el Brasil experimentó un aumento de 1,7 t a 2,3 t, convirtiéndose en el mayor poseedor de existencias de clonazepam en 2023. Las existencias en Italia también disminuyeron, de 900 kg en 2022 a 597 kg en 2023.

64. La importación mundial de clonazepam aumentó en forma constante hasta 2022, cuando alcanzó un máximo sin precedentes de 15,1 t. En 2023, sin embargo, las importaciones se redujeron a 11,4 t, en gran parte debido a las importaciones significativamente reducidas de Alemania (1,2 t, frente a 6,8 t en 2022) y Suiza (870 kg, frente a 1,2 t en 2022). En cambio, los Estados Unidos (1,2 t) y el Brasil (960 kg) comunicaron niveles de importación superiores a los de años anteriores. España no registró cambios significativos, con importaciones de 1,1 t en 2023, frente a 1,2 t en 2022.

65. En 2023, 89 países y territorios comunicaron datos de consumo de clonazepam, un aumento con respecto a los 78 de 2022. El Brasil (12,79 S-DDD$_{pmpd}$) registró el mayor consumo mundial, con un aumento significativo en comparación con las 6,53 S-DDD$_{pmpd}$ de 2022. México experimentó el aumento más sustancial, ya que el consumo pasó de 0,28 S-DDD$_{pmpd}$ en 2022 a 9,30 S-DDD$_{pmpd}$ en 2023. El Uruguay (8,05 S-DDD$_{pmpd}$) se mantuvo entre los países con mayor consumo declarado, a pesar de la disminución observada en comparación con las 14,08 S-DDD$_{pmpd}$ de 2022. El consumo en Chile pasó de 3,07 S-DDD$_{pmpd}$ a 7,77 S-DDD$_{pmpd}$. Entre 2022 y 2023, Costa Rica también informó de un aumento del consumo de 4,89 S-DDD$_{pmpd}$ a 7,22 S-DDD$_{pmpd}$, España comunicó una disminución de 8,12 S-DDD$_{pmpd}$ a 3,73 S-DDD$_{pmpd}$, y Portugal mostró un aumento de 2,38 S-DDD$_{pmpd}$ a 5,90 S-DDD$_{pmpd}$.

Alprazolam

66. El alprazolam, tranquilizante de acción rápida utilizado en el tratamiento a corto plazo de los trastornos de ansiedad, es una de las benzodiazepinas recetadas con más frecuencia en todo el mundo. En 2023, la fabricación mundial de esta sustancia alcanzó la cifra sin precedentes de 15,6 t, frente a las 12,8 t de 2022. La India aumentó sustancialmente su fabricación, de 6,9 t en 2022 a 10,8 t en 2023. Los Estados Unidos comunicaron una disminución de la fabricación de 2,7 t en 2022 a 2,1 t en 2023. Italia comunicó una fabricación total de 1,7 t, China informó de 513 kg y Australia, de 201 kg, mientras que otros países comunicaron cantidades menores. El total de las existencias mundiales de alprazolam disminuyó ligeramente, de 7,8 t en 2022 a 7,4 t en 2023, siendo los Estados Unidos (2,3 t), Italia (1,2 t), la India (797 kg) y China (745 kg) los países que poseían las mayores cantidades.

67. El volumen total de alprazolam importado a nivel mundial experimentó un fuerte aumento en 2023, cuando alcanzó las 14,9 t, frente a las 10,1 t de 2022. Un total de 139 países y territorios comunicaron importaciones en 2023. Israel experimentó un aumento significativo de las importaciones, que alcanzaron las 5,2 t, un incremento considerable respecto de los 8 kg registrados en 2022, que lo convierte en el mayor importador en 2023. Le siguieron los Estados Unidos, con 1,5 t, lo que supone un ligero aumento respecto a las 1,3 t de 2022. Italia también registró un aumento: importó 1,3 t, frente a los 664 kg de 2022. El Brasil importó 820 kg, frente a las 1,39 t de 2022. Suiza e Irlanda también registraron disminuciones, con importaciones de 504 kg y 399 kg, respectivamente. Otros países importaron cantidades más pequeñas.

68. En 2023, un total de 85 países y territorios proporcionaron datos sobre el consumo de alprazolam. De los países y territorios que comunicaron consumo, 11 notificaron tasas de consumo superiores a 10 S-DDD$_{pmpd}$ y otros 26 comunicaron tasas de entre 10 y 2 S-DDD$_{pmpd}$. De esos países y territorios, Hungría (51,02 S-DDD$_{pmpd}$), Australia (29,54 S-DDD$_{pmpd}$), Portugal (26,23 S-DDD$_{pmpd}$), España (21,24 S-DDD$_{pmpd}$) y Montenegro (20,73 S-DDD$_{pmpd}$) fueron los cinco principales consumidores de la sustancia en 2023.

Lorazepam

69. La fabricación mundial de lorazepam aumentó de 8,6 t en 2022 a 10,2 t en 2023. Este crecimiento fue impulsado principalmente por la India, donde la fabricación pasó de 1,8 t en 2022 a 3,1 t en 2023, y Alemania, que experimentó un aumento notable, de 954 kg en 2022 a 2,3 t en 2023. Por el contrario, Italia, aunque sigue siendo el mayor fabricante, registró una disminución de 5,4 t en 2022 a 4,3 t en 2023. Se fabricaron cantidades más pequeñas en China, Costa Rica y los Estados Unidos. Las existencias de los fabricantes aumentaron de 6,9 t en 2022 a 8,8 t en 2023. Alemania fue el mayor poseedor de reservas, con 2,6 t, seguida de Italia (1 t), el Reino de los Países Bajos (987 kg) y el Canadá (911 kg). Otros 35 países poseían cantidades más pequeñas.

70. En 2023, las importaciones mundiales de lorazepam alcanzaron un nuevo punto mínimo de 8,5 t, continuando su tendencia a la baja en comparación con las 8,6 t de 2022 y las 11,5 t de 2020. España fue el mayor importador en 2023, con 1,2 t, seguida de los Estados Unidos (1,2 t), Irlanda (741 kg), el Canadá (686 kg) y Alemania (657 kg). Las exportaciones mundiales de lorazepam siguieron una tendencia similar y alcanzaron las 9 t en 2023, lo que representa una disminución con respecto a las 9,6 t registradas en 2022. En 2023, las exportaciones de lorazepam volvieron a estar lideradas por Italia, que exportó 4,5 t. Alemania y la India también fueron exportadores importantes, con 1,6 t y 1,3 t, respectivamente. Estos tres países fueron los únicos que exportaron más de 1 t de lorazepam en 2023.

71. En 2023, comunicaron consumo de lorazepam 81 países y territorios, por encima de los 70 que lo habían hecho en 2022. Como en años anteriores, Portugal comunicó el mayor nivel de consumo de lorazepam, con 34,82 S-DDD_{pmpd}, seguido de España (26,92 S-DDD_{pmpd}), Montenegro (14,13 S-DDD_{pmpd}), Bélgica (12,92 S-DDD_{pmpd}) y Malta (11,98 S-DDD_{pmpd}). Además, otros 21 países notificaron niveles de consumo entre 2 y 10 S-DDD_{pmpd}. Los demás países y territorios declararon niveles de consumo inferiores a 2 S-DDD_{pmpd}.

Bromazepam

72. La fabricación de bromazepam alcanzó un máximo de 15,2 t en 2022 antes de disminuir a 9,0 t en 2023, cuando volvió a niveles más habitualmente observados en años anteriores. El pico de 2022 fue impulsado por Suiza, que comunicó 5,9 t tras no haber notificado la fabricación de la sustancia en 2021. En 2023, Suiza tampoco comunicó fabricación alguna de la sustancia. Italia siguió siendo el mayor fabricante en 2023, con 6,2 t. Los otros grandes fabricantes fueron la India (1,7 t) y el Brasil (1,1 t). En 2023, las existencias mundiales de bromazepam bajaron a 8,8 t, tras haber alcanzado un máximo de 11,6 t en 2022. Suiza redujo sustancialmente sus existencias, de 5,5 t en 2022 a 1,7 t en 2023. Italia aumentó sus existencias de 1,7 t en 2022 a 2,5 t en 2023, mientras que Francia experimentó una disminución, de 1,5 t a 1,2 t. El Brasil mantuvo unas existencias relativamente estables, con 1,2 t, un ligero descenso respecto a las 1,3 t de 2022.

73. En 2023, las importaciones mundiales de bromazepam aumentaron a 15,9 t, frente a las 13,1 t de 2022, impulsadas por un aumento significativo de las importaciones de Alemania, que aumentaron más del doble, de 1,9 t en 2022 a 4,5 t en 2023. Serbia, por su parte, registró una disminución de las importaciones, de 1,2 t a 893 kg. Otros importadores clave en 2023 fueron el Pakistán (1,7 t), Francia (1,6 t) e Italia (837 kg). Las exportaciones totales de bromazepam aumentaron de 13,7 t en 2022 a 16,3 t en 2023. Los exportadores principales en 2023 fueron Italia (5,8 t), Suiza (4,4 t), Alemania (3,2 t) y la India (1,7 t).

74. Los mayores consumidores de bromazepam en 2023 fueron Montenegro (15,47 S-DDD_{pmpd}) y Bosnia y Herzegovina (15,38 S-DDD_{pmpd}). Los otros países que registraron niveles de consumo superiores a 4 S-DDD_{pmpd} durante el año fueron Francia, con 5,43 S-DDD_{pmpd}, y Lituania, donde el consumo se mantuvo estable en 4,75 S-DDD_{pmpd}.

Clobazam

75. La fabricación de clobazam a nivel mundial disminuyó de 12,3 t en 2022 a 8,7 t en 2023. Esta disminución se debió principalmente a la ausencia de fabricación notificada por Francia, que había informado de 4,5 t el año anterior. En 2023, la India fue el principal fabricante a nivel mundial, con 6,6 t, seguida de Alemania, con 1,9 t. Italia, el Perú y los Estados Unidos comunicaron cantidades mucho menores.

76. Las importaciones mundiales de clobazam disminuyeron ligeramente, a 7,4 t en 2023, tras haber mantenido niveles relativamente estables de 7,5 t en 2022 y 7,9 t en 2021. La India fue el mayor importador de clobazam en 2023, con 1,2 t, seguida de Francia (999 kg), los Estados Unidos (792 kg), el Brasil (766 kg) e Indonesia (447 kg). Las exportaciones mundiales, que ascendieron a 8,2 t en 2023, también se mantuvieron sin cambios sustanciales respecto de su nivel de 2022. Francia (3,4 t), la India (2,5 t) y Alemania (1,5 t) fueron los únicos grandes exportadores de clobazam en 2023.

77. En 2023, comunicaron consumo de clobazam 66 países y territorios, frente a 55 en 2022. Portugal y Nueva Zelandia presentaron las tasas más elevadas, con 1,11 S-DDD_{pmpd} y 1,10 S-DDD_{pmpd}, respectivamente. Les siguió el Uruguay con 0,89 S-DDD_{pmpd}, mientras que el Canadá (0,83 S-DDD_{pmpd}) y Francia (0,73 S-DDD_{pmpd}) también registraron niveles de consumo considerables.

Clordiazepóxido

78. La fabricación mundial de clordiazepóxido ha aumentado, por lo general, en años recientes. Tras aumentar a 24,2 t en 2021 y alcanzar un máximo de 25,5 t en 2022, la fabricación mundial disminuyó a 22,8 t en 2023, debido principalmente a reducciones en Italia y la India. La fabricación comunicada por Italia disminuyó de 13,6 t en 2022 a 12,2 t en 2023, y la India comunicó una reducción de 11,3 t a 9,6 t. Al mismo tiempo, la fabricación de clordiazepóxido en China aumentó de 600 kg en 2022 a 978 kg en 2023. Las existencias de clordiazepóxido de los fabricantes aumentaron de 9,8 t en 2022 a 10,7 t en 2023 y se encontraban en 31 países, mayoritariamente en Italia (4,9 t), la India (1,4 t), los Estados Unidos (807 kg) y China (717 kg).

79. Las importaciones mundiales de clordiazepóxido han fluctuado en torno a las 13 t desde 2020. Tras un pico de 14,1 t en 2020, las importaciones disminuyeron a 13,9 t en 2022 y luego a 13 t en 2023. Suiza siguió siendo el mayor importador de la sustancia en 2023, con 6,2 t, seguida del Pakistán y Egipto, que importaron algo más de 1,2 t cada uno. Italia (12,4 t), Suiza (6,1 t) y la India (1,5 t) representaron más del 96 % del total de exportaciones de clordiazepóxido en 2023.

80. En 2023, 50 países y territorios comunicaron consumo de clordiazepóxido. Islandia registró el mayor nivel de consumo, con 1,29 S-DDD_{pmpd}, seguida de cerca por Portugal, con 1,20 S-DDD_{pmpd}. El Líbano (0,76 S-DDD_{pmpd}), Chile (0,70 S-DDD_{pmpd}) y Albania (0,63 S-DDD_{pmpd}) también comunicaron niveles de consumo significativos.

Oxazepam

81. La fabricación mundial de oxazepam ha seguido una tendencia a la baja desde que alcanzó un máximo de 27,5 t en 2019. Disminuyó a 22,8 t en 2020 y a 22,7 t en 2021, y luego continuó cayendo, a 19,9 t en 2022 y a 18,8 t en 2023. Esa tendencia a la baja puede atribuirse a la disminución de la producción en Italia, el principal fabricante, donde la fabricación notificada cayó de 27,3 t en 2019 a 15,3 t en 2023. La fabricación en la India, que ha experimentado fluctuaciones en los últimos años, cayó a 1,25 t en 2023. Al mismo tiempo, China, que había empezado a fabricar cantidades significativas en 2021, declaró 2,2 t en 2023. Del mismo modo, las existencias de oxazepam de los fabricantes han ido disminuyendo desde que alcanzaron un máximo de 32,7 t en 2020, cayendo a 21,4 t en 2022 y a 16,7 t en 2023. Había existencias de oxazepam en manos de los fabricantes en 24 países, con la mayoría comunicada por Francia (7 t), Italia (3,2 t), Austria (995 kg) y el Canadá (931 kg) para 2023.

82. Las importaciones mundiales de oxazepam han disminuido desde 2019, cuando alcanzaron un máximo de 30,5 t. Las importaciones cayeron a 26,9 t en 2020 y a 19,9 t en 2022 y 2023. Francia fue el mayor importador de oxazepam, con 9,7 t en 2023, frente a las 8,3 t de 2022. Le siguió Alemania, con 1,8 t, lo que supone un ligero aumento respecto a las 1,7 t del año anterior. Polonia también aumentó sus importaciones, a 1,6 t, y Sudáfrica importó 1,2 t en 2023. Italia (16,4 t), Alemania (1,4 t), Polonia (979 kg) y la India (959 kg) representaron el 97 % del total de exportaciones de oxazepam en 2023.

83. En 2023, 34 países comunicaron consumo de oxazepam. Francia comunicó el mayor nivel de consumo de oxazepam, con 9,24 S-DDD_{pmpd}, seguida de Islandia (5,63 S-DDD_{pmpd}), Noruega (4,66 S-DDD_{pmpd}), Finlandia (4,38 S-DDD_{pmpd}), Austria (3,53 S-DDD_{pmpd}), el Reino de los Países Bajos (3,30 S-DDD_{pmpd}), Portugal (2,29 S-DDD_{pmpd}), Suecia (2,16 S-DDD_{pmpd}) y Suiza (2,01 S-DDD_{pmpd}).

Español

Otras benzodiazepinas con una presencia destacada en el mercado lícito

84. Mientras que el alprazolam, el bromazepam, el clordiazepóxido, el clobazam, el clonazepam, el diazepam, el lorazepam, el midazolam y el oxazepam representan el 90 % de la fabricación lícita de benzodiazepinas que tienen una presencia destacada en el mercado lícito, el 10 % restante puede atribuirse a otras siete sustancias, a saber, nitrazepam, clorazepato, triazolam, temazepam, flunitrazepam, prazepam y flurazepam.

Nitrazepam

85. La fabricación de nitrazepam aumentó ligeramente a aproximadamente 2,9 t en 2023, frente a las 2,7 t registradas el año anterior. En 2023, Italia fue el principal fabricante, con 1,5 t, seguida de cerca por la India, que comunicó una fabricación total de 1,4 t. Las existencias continuaron su tendencia a la baja, pasando de 1,9 t en 2022 a 1,4 t en 2023. Italia poseía las mayores existencias (292 kg) en 2023, seguida de Francia (202 kg), y el resto estuvo distribuido entre otros 22 países. Las importaciones mundiales de la sustancia aumentaron a 2,0 t en 2023, con respecto a las 1,5 t de 2022. Del mismo modo, las exportaciones aumentaron de 1,6 t a 2,0 t. En 2023, 36 países informaron del consumo de nitrazepam; Malta fue el país que comunicó el nivel de consumo más elevado (1,98 S-DDD_{pmpd}).

Clorazepato

86. La fabricación mundial de clorazepato, en declive desde 2019, mostró un cambio de tendencia en 2023, cuando alcanzó 1,5 t, frente a los 794 kg de 2022. Italia fue el principal fabricante de la sustancia en 2023. Las existencias de la sustancia experimentaron un aumento significativo, de 1,5 t en 2022 a 6,6 t en 2023. Las importaciones mundiales de clorazepato también aumentaron considerablemente, de 4,4 t en 2022 a 8,3 t en 2023. Las exportaciones mundiales disminuyeron ligeramente en 2023, a 4,2 t. En 2023, 25 países informaron del consumo de clorazepato; España fue el país que comunicó el nivel de consumo más elevado (3,97 S-DDD_{pmpd}).

Triazolam

87. Tras un máximo de 1,1 t en 2021, la fabricación mundial de triazolam descendió a 252 kg en 2022 y a 58 kg en 2023, el segundo nivel más bajo desde que la sustancia se sometió a fiscalización internacional. Esta disminución se debió a una reducción significativa de la fabricación en los Estados Unidos y al hecho de que Italia no comunicó fabricación alguna. En 2023, la totalidad de la fabricación de esta sustancia correspondió a tres países: los Estados Unidos (31 kg), la India (22 kg) y la República de Corea (5 kg). Las existencias se redujeron en 75 kg y llegaron a 308 kg en 2023; la mayor parte estaba en manos de los Estados Unidos (156 kg), Italia (72 kg) e Irlanda (38 kg). Las importaciones y exportaciones de triazolam continuaron su tendencia a la baja en 2023. Las importaciones descendieron a 123 kg y las exportaciones, al mismo nivel, lo que supone una disminución con respecto a 2022, cuando ambas rondaron los 170 kg. En 2023, 26 países informaron del consumo de triazolam; Austria fue el país que comunicó el nivel de consumo más elevado (5,63 S-DDD_{pmpd}).

Temazepam

88. La fabricación de temazepam repuntó en 2023, a 6,9 t, desde su nivel más bajo en un decenio, que fue de 5,4 t en 2022. Sin embargo, el total para 2023 se mantuvo muy por debajo de las 11,6 t registradas en 2021. Italia volvió a ser el mayor fabricante de la sustancia en 2023, con un aumento de la fabricación hasta las 6,3 t. Le siguió la India, con 181 kg, mientras que Australia y Polonia comunicaron cantidades menores, a saber, 200 kg y 131 kg, respectivamente. En 2023, las existencias de temazepam se redujeron a 8,3 t, continuando su tendencia a la baja de los años anteriores, con la mayoría en manos de Italia (2,5 t) y de la India y el Canadá (que informaron de alrededor de 1 t cada una). Las importaciones totales notificadas de temazepam aumentaron ligeramente, de 7,7 t en 2022 a 8,2 t en 2023. Asimismo, el total de exportaciones aumentó a 8,5 t en 2023, con respecto a las 7,5 t de 2022. Con 4,08 S-DDD_{pmpd}, el Reino de los Países Bajos comunicó el nivel de consumo más elevado de los 19 países que facilitaron datos.

Flunitrazepam

89. La fabricación de flunitrazepam ha fluctuado considerablemente en los últimos años, ya que disminuyó de 2,2 t en 2020 a 36 kg en 2021 para luego aumentar a 182 kg en 2022 y a 544 kg en 2023. Italia fue el principal fabricante de esta sustancia en 2023, con 240 kg, seguida del Japón (165 kg) y la India (138 kg). Las existencias de flunitrazepam cayeron a 614 kg en 2023, en comparación con los 979 kg de 2022, y la mayor cantidad estaba en manos de Italia (193 kg). Las importaciones de la sustancia cayeron de 1,8 t en 2020 a 432 kg en 2022, pero luego subieron a 809 kg en 2023. Del mismo modo, las exportaciones mundiales de la sustancia cayeron de 1,9 t en 2020 a 530 kg en 2022 y aumentaron a 945 kg en 2023. El Uruguay comunicó el nivel más alto de consumo de flunitrazepam en 2023, 29,12 S-DDD$_{pmpd}$, casi el doble que en 2022. Otros 19 países y territorios comunicaron consumo de la sustancia.

Prazepam

90. La fabricación de prazepam aumentó significativamente en 2023, cuando alcanzó las 3,9 t, más del doble de las 1,7 t registradas en 2022, continuando la recuperación desde su mínimo de 850 kg en 2020. Italia fue el único país que fabricó la sustancia en 2023. Las existencias de prazepam aumentaron a 3,4 t en 2023, tras un descenso gradual de 7,1 t en 2018 a 2,4 t en 2022. Las existencias estaban en manos de 12 países. Las importaciones de prazepam aumentaron de 3,4 t en 2022 a 4 t en 2023. Asimismo, las exportaciones mostraron un leve aumento, de 3,5 t en 2022 a 3,7 t en 2023. En 2023, solo 13 países comunicaron consumo de prazepam, y el mayor nivel de consumo fue comunicado por Francia (2,07 S-DDD$_{pmpd}$).

Español

Flurazepam

91. La fabricación mundial de flurazepam repuntó hasta las 2,8 t en 2023, tras una importante caída en 2022, cuando solo se fabricaron 1,3 t, por debajo de las 3,4 t de 2021. El aumento se debió sobre todo a la recuperación de Italia, que declaró 2 t en 2023 tras haber fabricado solo 880 kg en 2022. Las existencias totales en 2023 ascendían a 2,3 t e Italia fue el país con la mayor cantidad (1 t). Las importaciones ascendieron a 1,7 t en 2023, lo que representa un aumento en comparación con las 1,5 t de 2022. Asimismo, las exportaciones aumentaron de 1,7 t en 2022 a 2,1 t en 2023. En 2023, 17 países comunicaron consumo de la sustancia y el mayor nivel de consumo fue notificado por España (0,92 S-DDD$_{pmpd}$).

Barbitúricos

92. En 2023, solo tres barbitúricos sometidos a fiscalización internacional tuvieron una presencia destacada en el mercado lícito (véase el cuadro 10). La fabricación de pentobarbital y barbital aumentó, interrumpiendo la tendencia a la baja de las últimas décadas. Al mismo tiempo, la fabricación de fenobarbital mantuvo su tendencia al alza y fue casi 10 t superior a la del año anterior. El amobarbital y el butalbital, que no figuran en el cuadro 10, siguen siendo objeto de fabricación y comercio en cantidades relativamente grandes.

Cuadro 10. Barbitúricos con una presencia destacada en el mercado lícito: fabricación e importación mundiales, por número de países y territorios importadores, 2023

Sustancia	*S-DDD (mg)*	*Fabricación (kg)*	*Importación (kg)*	*Número de países y territorios importadores*
Fenobarbital	100	374 079,15	208 219,59	158
Pentobarbital	100	58 630,12	61 852,59	68
Barbital	500	58 313,31	2 965,38	22

Fenobarbital

93. Tomando como base el peso bruto, el fenobarbital ha sido la sustancia sicotrópica sometida a fiscalización internacional que más se ha fabricado desde 2012. En 2023 se comunicó una fabricación total de 374 t de la sustancia, poco más de las 364,3 t notificadas en 2022. A pesar de un descenso de 46,8 t respecto al año anterior,

China siguió siendo el mayor fabricante de fenobarbital, con una producción de 174,9 t en 2023. La India, el otro gran fabricante de la sustancia, comunicó un total de 130,9 t en 2023, 31 t más que el año anterior. Hungría (42,2 t) y la Federación de Rusia (24,3 t) fueron los únicos otros países que comunicaron la fabricación de cantidades significativas en 2023.

94. Las existencias de fenobarbital en manos de los fabricantes aumentaron en 62,7 t, de 182,4 t en 2022 a 245,1 t en 2023. Las mayores existencias estaban en poder de China (67,9 t), seguida de la Federación de Rusia (49,4 t), Hungría (33,0 t) y el Brasil (26,0 t). Además, 12 países comunicaron existencias de entre 1 y 10,8 t, y otros 33 países comunicaron existencias inferiores a 1 t.

95. En 2023, 158 países y territorios comunicaron importaciones de fenobarbital, que pasa así a ser una de las sustancias sicotrópicas sometidas a fiscalización internacional con que más se comercia. Ese año, el volumen total de las importaciones mundiales ascendió a 208,2 t, lo que refleja una ligera disminución respecto de las 213 t importadas en 2022. El Brasil fue el país que importó mayores cantidades (41,2 t), seguido de la Federación de Rusia (23,0 t), los Estados Unidos (19,0 t), Suiza (10,0 t) y Dinamarca (8,9 t). Otros 22 países comunicaron importaciones de entre 1 y 6,8 t. Las importaciones notificadas por otros países y territorios variaron considerablemente, desde unas pocas docenas de gramos hasta varios cientos de kilogramos.

96. Las exportaciones totales de fenobarbital disminuyeron significativamente, de 226,8 t en 2022 a 199,8 t en 2023, en gran parte debido a una reducción significativa de las exportaciones de China, el segundo mayor exportador en 2023. Las exportaciones de fenobarbital del país cayeron de 86,1 t en 2022 a 59,8 t en 2023. Los otros principales exportadores en 2023 fueron, en primer lugar, la India (79,0 t), seguida de Hungría (20,7 t), Suiza (9,7 t), Dinamarca (9,1 t), Alemania (5,2 t), Croacia (3,1 t), Francia (2,7 t), el Reino de los Países Bajos (2,4 t), Rumanía (2,3 t) y Kenya (1,5 t).

97. El número de países y territorios que proporcionaron datos sobre el consumo de fenobarbital aumentó de 89 en 2022 a 101 en 2023. En la figura 13 se muestra una comparación regional del número de países y territorios que proporcionaron datos de consumo de 2019 a 2023. Durante ese período, el número de países y territorios que proporcionaron datos sobre el consumo de fenobarbital se mantuvo constantemente alto en las Américas y en Europa. En cifras absolutas, Oceanía fue la región en que menos países y territorios proporcionaron esos datos cada año. El número de países y territorios de Asia que proporcionaron datos aumentó considerablemente en 2023, cuando cinco países más comunicaron datos, mientras que el número correspondiente en África solo experimentó un ligero aumento.

98. Entre los países y territorios que proporcionaron datos, el Brasil comunicó la tasa de consumo de fenobarbital más elevada de 2023 (4,96 S-DDD_{pmpd}), muy poco más que el año anterior (4,95 S-DDD_{pmpd}). En Europa, San Marino (2,17 S-DDD_{pmpd}) fue el mayor consumidor, seguido de Francia (1,28 S-DDD_{pmpd}) y Montenegro (1,24 S-DDD_{pmpd}). En África, Seychelles comunicó la mayor tasa de consumo (4,81 S-DDD_{pmpd}), mientras que Burkina Faso notificó la tasa más baja (0,01 S-DDD_{pmpd}). La disparidad intrarregional en las Américas también fue grande; como se señaló anteriormente, el Brasil (4,96 S-DDD_{pmpd}) comunicó el mayor nivel de consumo en 2023, mientras que Cuba comunicó el más bajo (menos de 0,03 S-DDD_{pmpd}). En Asia, los niveles de consumo entre los países y territorios que proporcionaron datos también fueron muy dispares: China comunicó la mayor tasa de consumo (2,48 S-DDD_{pmpd}) y el Iraq, la menor (0,003 S-DDD_{pmpd}). En Oceanía, siete países y territorios proporcionaron datos sobre el consumo de fenobarbital, de los cuales Australia notificó la tasa de consumo más elevada (0,85 S-DDD_{pmpd}).

99. En el sitio web de la JIFE puede encontrarse información más detallada sobre el consumo de fenobarbital.

Figura 13. Fenobarbital: número de países y territorios que comunicaron consumo, por región, 2019–2023

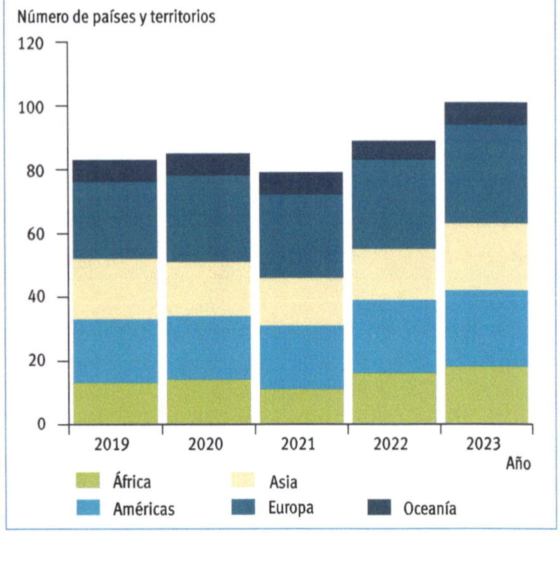

Pentobarbital

100. Los Estados Unidos y Alemania, que una vez más fueron los principales fabricantes de pentobarbital en 2023, comunicaron la fabricación de 33,6 t y 24,6 t, respectivamente. El Japón comunicó un aumento significativo de su fabricación de esta sustancia, de 0,5 kg (2022) a 353 kg (2023). En total, se fabricaron 58,6 t de pentobarbital en 2023, lo que constituyó un leve aumento respecto de las 56,0 t comunicadas en 2022. La fabricación tanto en Alemania como en los Estados Unidos se mantuvo prácticamente sin cambios en 2023 en comparación con el año anterior. La India y Suiza también comunicaron la fabricación de la sustancia, pero en cantidades de apenas unos gramos cada una.

101. Las existencias de pentobarbital en manos de los fabricantes aumentaron de 43,0 t en 2022 a 55,6 t en 2023. Los Estados Unidos tenían unas 16,8 t de existencias y Alemania comunicó 16,7 t, seguida del Reino de los Países Bajos (8,0 t), Dinamarca (3,4 t), Francia (3,3 t), Austria (2,4 t), Suiza y el Reino Unido (1,2 t cada uno). Otros 16 países notificaron existencias, que en cada caso no excedieron de unos pocos cientos de kilogramos.

102. A la cabeza de las importaciones de pentobarbital estuvo el Reino de los Países Bajos, que comunicó 16,5 t en 2023, lo que representó un aumento de 4,7 t con respecto a las 11,8 t que había importado en 2022. La mayor parte de las importaciones de ese país se destinó a la reexportación. Las importaciones de pentobarbital comunicadas por otros países no variaron mucho con respecto a los años anteriores; los otros principales importadores fueron Dinamarca (7,0 t) y Alemania (6,6 t). Otros 8 países comunicaron importaciones de más de 1 t y otros 18 países, de entre 100 kg y 1 t, mientras que el resto de los países notificó cantidades que iban de unos pocos gramos a varias docenas de kilogramos cada uno.

103. Las exportaciones mundiales de pentobarbital también aumentaron a 47,5 t en 2023, frente a 41,5 t en 2022. Como principal fabricante de pentobarbital, Alemania también se situó a la cabeza de las exportaciones de esa sustancia, con 22,3 t en 2023, cifra ligeramente inferior a las 23,0 t comunicadas en 2022. El Reino de los Países Bajos fue el segundo mayor exportador, con 11,8 t, lo que constituyó una ligera disminución con respecto a los años anteriores. Dinamarca y Austria exportaron más de 5,1 t y 3,4 t, respectivamente.

104. Para 2023, un total de 44 países y territorios proporcionaron datos sobre el consumo de pentobarbital, lo que representa un aumento con respecto a los 38 que lo habían hecho en 2022. Luxemburgo comunicó la mayor tasa de consumo de la sustancia en 2023 con 4,12 $S\text{-}DDD_{pmpd}$, nivel ligeramente inferior a las 4,14 $S\text{-}DDD_{pmpd}$ de 2022. Dinamarca y Australia fueron los únicos otros países que comunicaron un consumo superior a 3 $S\text{-}DDD_{pmpd}$.

Barbital

105. La fabricación mundial de barbital aumentó de 48,6 t en 2022 a 58,3 t en 2023, superando el máximo anterior de 57,9 t comunicado para 2019. China siguió siendo el principal fabricante, con 36,8 t fabricadas en 2023, lo que representó un aumento respecto de las 30,6 t fabricadas en 2022. Los únicos otros países que comunicaron fabricación de barbital en 2023 fueron la India (20,0 t), Alemania (1,1 t) y el Japón (341 kg). Los niveles de fabricación en esos países no cambiaron significativamente con respecto al año anterior, excepto en la India, donde la cantidad comunicada aumentó de 13 t a 20 t. Las existencias de barbital de los fabricantes ascendieron a 46,8 t en 2023, un aumento significativo en comparación con las 29,1 t notificadas para 2022. China poseía 40,7 t de la sustancia, casi el 87 % de las existencias mundiales y casi el doble de la cifra comunicada para 2022, mientras que Alemania (4,3 t) y Francia (812 kg) tenían la mayor parte de la cantidad restante.

106. El comercio de barbital fue algo limitado, ya que solo 22 países y territorios comunicaron importaciones de esa sustancia. Las importaciones totales para 2023 ascendieron a algo menos de 3 t, 234 kg por encima de las 2,7 t comunicadas para 2022. El mayor importador de barbital en 2023 fueron los Estados Unidos (1,2 t), seguidos de Francia (742,4 kg), Tailandia (712,7 kg), Suiza (166,8 kg) y el Reino Unido (97,5 kg). Las exportaciones totales de la sustancia se redujeron en solo 26 kg, a 2,6 t en 2023, y Alemania (1,9 t) concentró la mayor parte de las exportaciones mundiales. El Japón (357,6 kg) y Suiza (187,5 kg) fueron los únicos otros países que comunicaron haber exportado cantidades considerables de la sustancia.

107. En cuanto al consumo de barbital, se dispone de datos de relativamente pocos países. Solo 16 países proporcionaron datos de consumo correspondientes a 2023 y, excepto China (0,06 S-DDD$_{pmpd}$), todos ellos comunicaron niveles de consumo inferiores a 0,01 S-DDD$_{pmpd}$.

Otros sedantes hipnóticos

108. En la actualidad, de los ocho sedantes hipnóticos que no son ni benzodiazepinas ni barbitúricos, solo dos son objeto de comercio lícito: el GHB y el zolpidem. Es necesario ejercer cautela al extraer conclusiones a partir de las estadísticas sobre el GHB, ya que la S-DDD de esa sustancia es actualmente de 7.500 mg, muy superior a la de cualquier otra sustancia sicotrópica sujeta a fiscalización internacional. Dado que los valores de la S-DDD de la mayoría de las sustancias fiscalizadas con arreglo al Convenio de 1971 se sitúan entre 1 y 200 mg, podría parecer que las cifras brutas relativas a la fabricación o el comercio de GHB indican que la sustancia es muy común en el mercado. En realidad, el elevado valor de la S-DDD del GHB se debe a que la sustancia ha de fabricarse en cantidades entre decenas y cientos de veces mayores que otras sustancias sicotrópicas para alcanzar niveles de dosificación equivalentes. Esto puede apreciarse en el cuadro 11, en que el peso base de una dosis diaria definida con fines estadísticos de GHB es 750 veces mayor que el del zolpidem.

Cuadro 11. Otros sedantes hipnóticos con una presencia destacada en el mercado lícito: fabricación y número de países y territorios importadores, por fabricación medida en S-DDD, 2023

Sustancia	*S-DDD (mg)*	*Fabricación (kg)*	*Fabricación (millones de S-DDD)*	*Número de países y territorios importadores*
Zolpidem	10	40 740,39	4 074,04	118
Ácido *gamma*-hidroxibutírico	7 500	57 789,12	7,71	43

Ácido *gamma*-hidroxibutírico

109. Debido a su alto valor de S-DDD, el GHB debe fabricarse en cantidades mucho mayores que otras sustancias para satisfacer su demanda mundial con fines médicos y científicos, aunque no es objeto de un comercio tan extenso como el de otras sustancias sicotrópicas sujetas a fiscalización internacional.

110. Para 2023 se comunicó una fabricación de 57,8 t de GHB, lo que representa un aumento considerable respecto de las 51,9 t notificadas para 2022. Ese aumento se debió principalmente al hecho de que Irlanda no comunicó fabricación alguna de la sustancia en 2021, pero reanudó la fabricación en 2022 y 2023. Irlanda (26,2 t) fue la principal fabricante de GHB en 2023, seguida de los Estados Unidos (15,0 t) y la India (9,8 t). Las existencias de GHB en manos de los fabricantes aumentaron drásticamente, de 119,7 t en 2022 a 217,0 t en 2023. El país que poseía las mayores existencias era Irlanda, que comunicó algo más de 61,9 t; le siguieron los Estados Unidos (20,8 t), Francia (6,5 t), Ucrania (3,5 t), Italia (3,0 t) y Alemania (2,8 t). Suiza comunicó un fuerte descenso de sus existencias de la sustancia, que disminuyeron de 2,5 t en 2021 a 207,9 kg en 2023 debido a las exportaciones.

111. En 2023, 43 países y territorios comunicaron importaciones de GHB, que ascendieron a un total de 62,9 t, lo que refleja una disminución importante en comparación con las 78,1 t notificadas por 41 países en 2022. En 2023, los Estados Unidos comunicaron la mayor cantidad de importaciones (35,8 t), seguidos de Francia (4,6 t), Italia (4,1 t), Bélgica (4,0 t), Letonia (2,7 t), la Federación de Rusia (2,0 t) e Irlanda (1,7 t). Otros tres países comunicaron importaciones de GHB de más de 1 t, mientras que el resto de los países y territorios notificaron cantidades menores.

112. Las exportaciones de GHB se situaron en 63,3 t en 2023, por debajo de las 76,4 t notificadas en 2022. El descenso puede atribuirse sobre todo a las importantes disminuciones de las exportaciones de Irlanda, que pasó de 42,5 t en 2022 a 32,5 t en 2023, pero siguió siendo el principal exportador de la sustancia. A Irlanda le siguieron los Estados Unidos (7,1 t), Alemania (6,4 t), la India (4,1 t), Francia (4,0 t), Bélgica (3,0 t), Letonia (2,6 t) y el Reino Unido (1,5 t), y otros cinco países comunicaron exportaciones de GHB de entre 100 kg y 1 t.

113. En 2023, notificaron consumo de GHB sobre todo países de Europa, además del Canadá y los Estados Unidos, por lo que se mantiene la tendencia de los dos últimos años. La tasa de consumo más elevada fue la comunicada por los Estados Unidos (0,04 S-DDD_{pmpd}). Italia, Noruega, el Reino de los Países Bajos y Suecia comunicaron tasas de consumo de 0,02 S-DDD_{pmpd}, mientras que otros países que proporcionaron datos de consumo comunicaron niveles inferiores a esa cifra.

Zolpidem

114. El zolpidem es una de las sustancias sicotrópicas sujetas a fiscalización internacional con las que más se comercia. En 2023, 118 países y territorios informaron de que habían importado la sustancia y en todas las regiones del mundo se comunicó el consumo de zolpidem.

115. La fabricación de zolpidem aumentó ligeramente, de 39,1 t en 2022 a 40,7 t en 2023. Como en años anteriores, la India fue el principal fabricante de la sustancia, con 25,8 t en 2023, lo que representa un aumento de 4,6 t con respecto a 2022. Chequia fue el segundo mayor fabricante en 2023, con 7,6 t, por encima de las 0,4 t comunicadas en 2022. Tras haber notificado la fabricación de 4,2 t en 2022, el Brasil comunicó 3,1 t en 2023. El Japón (2,6 t) y la Argentina (1 t) también fueron importantes fabricantes de zolpidem en 2023. Francia, que había comunicado 3,5 t en 2022, no comunicó fabricación alguna de la sustancia en 2023.

116. Las existencias mundiales de zolpidem en posesión de los fabricantes prácticamente se quintuplicaron, de 18,4 t en 2022 a 87,9 t en 2023. La mayor cantidad correspondió a Francia (16,2 t), seguida de Sudáfrica (6,7 t), el Brasil (4,4 t), la India (3,1 t) y Chequia (3,0 t). Otros 33 países poseían cantidades menores.

117. Las importaciones totales de zolpidem aumentaron de 25,5 t en 2022 a 35,8 t en 2023. Como en años anteriores, los Estados Unidos comunicaron las mayores importaciones de zolpidem, con 4,9 t, lo que representa una disminución respecto de las 6,4 t comunicadas en 2022. El Brasil (3,9 t), España (3,0 t), Alemania (2,9 t), el Japón (1,6 t), Polonia (1,6 t) y la Argentina (1,5 t) fueron los otros principales importadores de la sustancia. Varios de esos países importaron zolpidem con fines de reexportación.

118. El total de exportaciones de zolpidem se ha mantenido relativamente estable durante varios años. En 2023, el total de las exportaciones comunicadas ascendió a 37,6 t, una disminución moderada respecto de las 41,6 t que se habían exportado en 2022, cantidad que, a su vez, había sido superior a las 37,3 t comunicadas para 2021. Como mayor fabricante de zolpidem, la India fue el principal exportador de la sustancia en 2023, con 13,6 t, una disminución frente a las 18,1 t comunicadas para 2022. Otros importantes exportadores fueron Chequia (7,7 t) y Francia (5,4 t). Alemania, España, el Reino de los Países Bajos y Serbia declararon exportaciones de aproximadamente entre 1 t y 2 t cada uno.

119. En 2023, el número total de países y territorios que proporcionaron datos sobre el consumo de zolpidem aumentó en 8, con lo que se llegó al total de 73 (véase la figura 14). A nivel regional, se observó un aumento de las notificaciones en todas las regiones. Europa fue la única región en la que más de la mitad de los países y territorios proporcionaron datos de consumo.

120. En 2023, Bosnia y Herzegovina comunicó el mayor consumo de zolpidem de todo el mundo, con 91,03 S-DDD_{pmpd}, seguida de Chequia, con 16,74 S-DDD_{pmpd}. En general, en los países y territorios que proporcionaron datos, el consumo medio de zolpidem en Europa fue significativamente mayor que en otras regiones. En África, Marruecos (0,54 S-DDD_{pmpd}) comunicó el mayor nivel de consumo, mientras que Angola (0,002 S-DDD_{pmpd}) comunicó el menor. En las Américas, el Brasil comunicó el

Figura 14. Zolpidem: número de países y territorios que comunicaron consumo, por región, 2019–2023

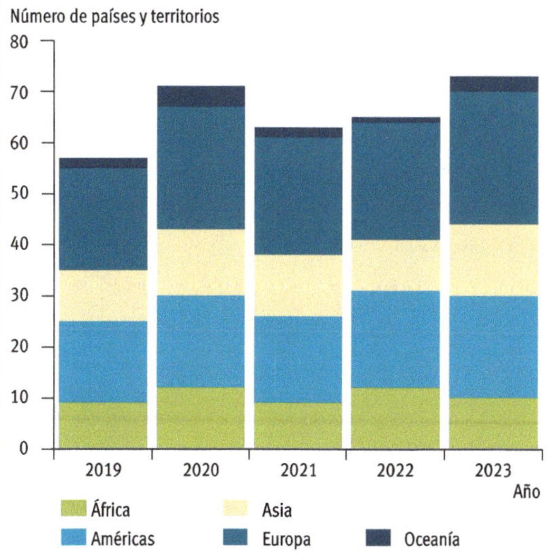

nivel de consumo más elevado (7,160 $S\text{-}DDD_{pmpd}$) y el Ecuador, el más bajo (0,01 $S\text{-}DDD_{pmpd}$). En Asia, la República de Corea comunicó el mayor nivel de consumo (8,96 $S\text{-}DDD_{pmpd}$) y Maldivas, el menor (0,04 $S\text{-}DDD_{pmpd}$). En Oceanía, Australia comunicó el nivel de consumo más elevado (0,97 $S\text{-}DDD_{pmpd}$), mientras que los Estados Federados de Micronesia comunicaron el nivel más bajo (0,002 $S\text{-}DDD_{pmpd}$).

Meprobamato

121. El meprobamato, sustancia de la Lista IV del Convenio de 1971, es el único ansiolítico no benzodiazepínico sometido a fiscalización internacional que tiene actualmente una presencia destacada en el mercado lícito. Aunque solo se comercializa en aproximadamente una docena de países, en cuanto a peso bruto es una de las sustancias sicotrópicas sujetas a fiscalización internacional que más se fabrican.

Cuadro 12. Meprobamato: fabricación e importación mundiales y número de países importadores, 2023

Sustancia	*S-DDD (mg)*	*Fabricación (kg)*	*Importación (kg)*	*Número de países importadores*
Meprobamato	1 200	39 535,67	49 194,72	14

122. Si bien la fabricación y el comercio se limitan a un grupo pequeño de países, el elevado peso de la dosis de meprobamato, como en el caso del GHB, requiere que se fabriquen cantidades importantes de la sustancia para satisfacer la demanda. Como se muestra en el cuadro 12, en 2023 se fabricaron 39,5 t de meprobamato, lo que representa una disminución considerable respecto de las 97,1 t comunicadas en 2022. Como en años anteriores, en 2023 China y la India fueron los principales fabricantes de la sustancia y notificaron 26,0 t y 13,5 t, respectivamente. Las existencias mundiales de meprobamato en manos de los fabricantes ascendieron a 49,2 t en 2023, un aumento considerable en comparación con la cantidad comunicada en 2022 (37 t). China tenía las mayores existencias (40,6 t), seguida de Sudáfrica (3,8 t). La India y el Líbano también poseían importantes existencias de la sustancia en 2023, con 1,9 t y 1,2 t, respectivamente.

123. Las importaciones totales de meprobamato en 2023 ascendieron a 49,2 t, lo que representa un aumento de 4,4 t con respecto a las 44,8 t comunicadas en 2022. Sudáfrica concentró más de la mitad de las importaciones de la sustancia (26,4 t), seguida de la India (15,8 t) y la República Democrática del Congo (3,8 t). Las exportaciones de meprobamato cayeron de 114,4 t en 2022 a 41,0 t en 2023. La India y China, principales fabricantes de la sustancia, lideraron también las exportaciones, con 21,7 t y 17,7 t, respectivamente.

124. Puesto que la fabricación y el comercio de meprobamato se limitan a un pequeño grupo de países, el consumo de la sustancia también ha sido muy limitado. En 2023, solo 3 países proporcionaron datos sobre el consumo de la sustancia, lo que representa una disminución con respecto a los 13 que lo hicieron en 2022. El mayor nivel de consumo en 2023 lo registró el Líbano, con 0,21 $S\text{-}DDD_{pmpd}$, seguido de Bélgica (0,02 $S\text{-}DDD_{pmpd}$) y la India (0,01 $S\text{-}DDD_{pmpd}$).

Buprenorfina

125. De los tres analgésicos incluidos en la Lista III del Convenio de 1971, solo una sustancia, la buprenorfina, tuvo una presencia destacada en el mercado lícito en 2023. Ese año, 97 países y territorios importaron buprenorfina, opioide utilizado principalmente como analgésico y en el tratamiento de la dependencia de los opioides (véase el cuadro 13).

Cuadro 13. Buprenorfina: fabricación e importación mundiales y número de países y territorios importadores, 2023

Sustancia	*S-DDD (mg)*	*Fabricación (kg)*	*Importación (kg)*	*Número de países y territorios importadores*
Buprenorfina	8	15 537,57	9 915,08	97

126. La fabricación mundial de buprenorfina comenzó a aumentar gradualmente a finales de la década de 1990, cuando la sustancia empezó a utilizarse en mayores dosis para el tratamiento del dolor y la adicción a los opioides.

Tras un importante descenso en 2010, la fabricación mundial comunicada de la sustancia aumentó constantemente hasta alcanzar las 17,2 t en 2018, pero disminuyó a 10,5 t en 2019 debido a que el Reino Unido, principal fabricante de la sustancia hasta ese momento, no comunicó fabricación alguna. En 2023, la fabricación total alcanzó las 15,5 t y cuatro países comunicaron la fabricación de cantidades destacables de la sustancia, a saber, el Reino Unido (5,9 t), Alemania (2,6 t), los Estados Unidos (2,6 t) y la India (2,2 t).

127. El comercio de buprenorfina disminuyó de 13,5 t de importaciones en 2022 a 9,9 t en 2023. Como ya se ha señalado, comunicaron importaciones 97 países y territorios de todo el mundo, y el principal importador fueron los Estados Unidos (6,6 t), seguidos de Francia (642,2 kg), Alemania (484,4 kg), el Reino Unido (272,6 kg) y el Canadá (246,9 kg). Otros tres países importaron aproximadamente 100 kg cada uno. En cuanto a las exportaciones, el Reino Unido (5,3 t), Alemania (1,6 t), y Chequia (1,3 t) fueron los principales exportadores en 2023.

128. En 2023, 64 países y territorios proporcionaron datos sobre el consumo de buprenorfina. Se comunicó consumo de la sustancia principalmente en Europa y América del Norte, al igual que en años anteriores (véase el cuadro 14). En 2023, la tasa de consumo más elevada fue la notificada por los Estados Unidos (8,84 S-DDD_{pmpd}), seguidos de Islandia (3,60 S-DDD_{pmpd}), el Reino Unido (2,45 S-DDD_{pmpd}), Finlandia (2,25 S-DDD_{pmpd}) y Australia y Montenegro (2,11 S-DDD_{pmpd} en ambos casos). Australia proporcionó datos sobre el consumo de buprenorfina por primera vez en 2023.

Cuadro 14. Buprenorfina: tasas de consumo en determinados países y territorios, en orden descendente según el nivel de consumo, 2021–2023

	S-DDD por cada 1.000 habitantes por día		
País o territorio	*2021*	*2022*	*2023*
Estados Unidos	9,17	9,16	8,84
Islandia	1,52	9,53	3,60
Reino Unido	3,30	2,13	2,45
Finlandia	2,05	2,10	2,25
Australia	–	–	2,11
Montenegro	2,21	2,10	2,11
Canadá	1,92	2,01	2,10
Noruega	–	1,98	1,97
Portugal	0,47	1,48	1,69
Suecia	1,55	1,59	1,64
Francia	–	–	1,48
Gibraltar	0,16	0,11	1,43
Austria	1,26	1,25	1,22
Alemania	1,26	1,66	1,01
Polonia	0,72	0,70	0,90

Preparados exentos

129. Las obligaciones previstas en el artículo 16 del Convenio de 1971 respecto de la presentación de informes exigen que las partes comuniquen las cantidades de sustancias sicotrópicas utilizadas para la fabricación de otras sustancias sicotrópicas, de preparados exentos y de sustancias no sicotrópicas. Estos usos de sustancias sicotrópicas son distintos del consumo notificado de cantidades utilizadas con fines médicos y científicos.

130. El artículo 3 del Convenio de 1971 autoriza a los países a eximir de la aplicación de algunas medidas de fiscalización a los preparados que contienen sustancias sicotrópicas. Solo pueden quedar exentos los preparados que contengan sustancias incluidas en las Listas II, III o IV del Convenio. Gracias a esas exenciones, los países pueden facilitar la disponibilidad de ciertos medicamentos en su territorio o el comercio de estos.

131. En 2023 se utilizaron cinco sustancias de la Lista II en cantidades de 0,01 kg o superiores para fabricar preparados exentos (véase el cuadro 15). No se notificó el uso de levometanfetamina. En años anteriores, los

Español

Estados Unidos habían sido el único país que comunicó la utilización de levometanfetamina para fabricar preparados exentos. Alemania fue el único país que informó de la utilización de GHB para la fabricación de preparados exentos en 2023, siguiendo la tendencia observada desde 2019. Azerbaiyán comunicó el uso de metanfetamina para fabricar preparados exentos por primera vez en 2023 y fue el único país que lo hizo. En 2023, Hungría comunicó el uso de 1,38 t de racemato de metanfetamina. Australia comunicó casi la totalidad de la utilización de *delta*-9-THC para preparados exentos en 2023. Además, los Estados Unidos utilizaron menos de 0,01 kg de dexanfetamina para preparados exentos.

Cuadro 15. Sustancias de la Lista II utilizadas para la fabricación de preparados exentos, por cantidad utilizada, 2021–2023

	Cantidad utilizada (kg)		
Sustancia	*2021*	*2022*	*2023*
Racemato de metanfetamina	0,03	127,49	1 388,89
Metanfetamina	0,05	0,01	412,00
Ácido *gamma*-hidroxibutírico	139,18	71,89	216,99
delta-9-Tetrahidrocannabinol	8,96	25,51	8,85
Dexanfetamina	0,01	0,05	0,01
Metacualona	<0,01	<0,01	<0,01
Metilfenidato	<0,01	–	<0,01
Fenciclidina (PCP)	<0,01	–	<0,01
Anfetamina	0,01	0,01	<0,01
Secobarbital	0,02	<0,01	–
3,4-Metilendioxipirovalerona (MDPV)	0,00	–	–
N-Bencilpiperazina	–	0,01	–
CUMIL-PEGACLONE	5,41	–	–
Etilona	–	<0,01	–
Levanfetamina	–	<0,01	–
Levometanfetamina	178,02	247,25	–

132. Según los datos correspondientes a 2023, en ese año se utilizó una sustancia incluida en la Lista III en una cantidad de 0,01 kg o superior para fabricar preparados exentos (véase el cuadro 16). Desde 2017, los Estados Unidos han sido el único país que ha comunicado el uso de butalbital en la fabricación de preparados exentos. La mayor parte del butalbital fabricado por los Estados Unidos se utiliza para fabricar esos preparados, como el fosfato de codeína y el acetaminofeno, u otras sustancias no sicotrópicas. El uso de buprenorfina para preparados exentos ha seguido disminuyendo desde 2020 y en 2022 solo se utilizó una cantidad insignificante. En 2023 no se notificó ningún uso de buprenorfina con este fin.

Cuadro 16. Sustancias de la Lista III utilizadas para la fabricación de preparados exentos, por cantidad utilizada, 2021–2023

	Cantidad utilizada (kg)		
Sustancia	*2021*	*2022*	*2023*
Butalbital	7 584,69	5 303,81	978,69
Buprenorfina	1,45	0,01	–
Pentobarbital	<0,01	<0,01	<0,01
Amobarbital	<0,01	–	<0,01

133. Doce países comunicaron la utilización de 17 sustancias de la Lista IV del Convenio de 1971 en cantidades de 0,01 kg o superiores para la fabricación de preparados exentos en 2023 (véase el cuadro 17). En general, las tendencias en la fabricación de preparados exentos se han mantenido prácticamente sin cambios en los últimos años. La Federación de Rusia y Ucrania han concentrado la mayor parte del fenobarbital destinado a los

preparados exentos. Sin embargo, Argelia comunicó por primera vez el uso de más de 1 t de fenobarbital para tales fines en 2022. La utilización para la fabricación de preparados exentos de la mayor parte de las benzodiazepinas que figuran en el cuadro 17 y casi todo el zolpidem y el oxazepam se concentraron en Alemania.

Cuadro 17. Sustancias de la Lista IV utilizadas para la fabricación de preparados exentos, por cantidad utilizada, 2021–2023

	Cantidad utilizada (kg)		
Sustancia	*2021*	*2022*	*2023*
Fenobarbital	17 956,20	18 049,26	61 380,65
Diazepam	2 408,39	1 597,26	1 918,90
Zolpidem	1 897,51	1 790,10	1 811,52
Oxazepam	2 377,52	1 405,61	1 680,15
Barbital	1 615,36	1 531,50	1 001,14
Temazepam	410,04	594,15	516,09
Bromazepam	609,38	513,54	515,04
Prazepam	312,00	211,88	311,80
Clordiazepóxido	93,96	218,54	197,60
Midazolam	277,62	228,28	183,37
Flurazepam	197,44	–	148,08
Lorazepam	224,94	85,69	94,44
Clonazepam	48,47	23,42	44,08
Alprazolam	32,69	43,47	33,72
Nitrazepam	59,03	18,00	26,00
Lormetazepam	37,66	3,63	11,43
Fentermina	8,21	0,01	0,01
Nordazepam	<0,01	<0,01	<0,01
Triazolam	–	–	<0,01
Flubromazolam	4,99	–	–

SISTEMA MUNDIAL DE PREVISIONES DE SUSTANCIAS SICOTRÓPICAS PARA FINES MÉDICOS Y CIENTÍFICOS Y TENDENCIAS RECIENTES

Sistema de previsiones de sustancias sicotrópicas y adhesión a este por los países

Introducción

134. Quienes redactaron el Convenio de 1971 no incorporaron un sistema de previsiones para las sustancias sicotrópicas similar al establecido para los estupefacientes fiscalizados con arreglo a la Convención de 1961 en su forma enmendada. Solamente después de la entrada en vigor del Convenio de 1971, la comunidad internacional determinó que se necesitaba un sistema mundial para que los países pudieran indicar sus necesidades anuales de sustancias sicotrópicas, evitar el exceso de oferta y prevenir la desviación de esas sustancias del comercio internacional.

135. En sus resoluciones 1981/7 y 1991/44, el Consejo Económico y Social invitó a los países a que comunicaran periódicamente a la Junta las previsiones de sus necesidades anuales de sustancias incluidas en las Listas II, III y IV del Convenio de 1971 para fines médicos y científicos. En el caso de las sustancias de la Lista I no se requieren esas previsiones. Desde la aprobación de esas resoluciones, la JIFE ha recibido previsiones de diferentes países y territorios y las ha puesto a disposición de la comunidad internacional por diversos medios. El sistema se ha convertido en un pilar fundamental de la fiscalización del movimiento internacional de sustancias sicotrópicas.

136. Desde que se adoptó el sistema de previsiones, la Junta ha aconsejado a los países que presenten, al menos cada tres años, previsiones actualizadas de sus necesidades anuales lícitas de sustancias sicotrópicas. Además, se invita a los países a que presenten cualquier modificación de sus previsiones de sustancias específicas cuando sea necesario, por ejemplo, si sus necesidades de una sustancia superan una previsión establecida anteriormente.

Presentación de las previsiones y adhesión al sistema de previsiones de sustancias sicotrópicas

137. Por lo general, los países y territorios se adhieren al sistema de previsiones de sustancias sicotrópicas, a pesar de que este se estableció fuera del ámbito de aplicación del Convenio de 1971 y es totalmente voluntario. Todos los países y territorios reconocidos por las Naciones Unidas han presentado previsiones al menos para algunas de las sustancias sometidas a fiscalización en virtud del Convenio. En el caso de que un país no haya establecido o no pueda establecer sus propias previsiones, la Junta lo hará para garantizar que ese país pueda importar las sustancias sicotrópicas más esenciales. En años recientes, el único país para el que la Junta ha tenido que establecer previsiones fue Sudán del Sur, en 2011.

138. Una vez establecidas, las previsiones de sustancias sicotrópicas no pierden validez y, por tanto, no es preciso que los países y territorios las actualicen anualmente, a diferencia de lo que ocurre con los estupefacientes sometidos a fiscalización en virtud de la Convención de 1961 en su forma enmendada. No obstante, se recomienda a los países y territorios que actualicen sus previsiones cada tres años para asegurarse de que estas reflejan adecuadamente sus necesidades médicas y científicas. Por ello, no todos los países y territorios presentan previsiones nuevas cada año y, si consideran que sus necesidades están cubiertas, tal vez no modifiquen las previsiones que ya hayan establecido.

139. Cada año numerosos países y territorios facilitan a la Junta previsiones actualizadas de determinadas sustancias sicotrópicas. En el período comprendido entre 2014 y 2023, entre 90 y 104 países y territorios proporcionaron un total de entre 2.690 y 3.700 previsiones de sustancias sicotrópicas cada año (véase el cuadro 18). Durante el mismo período, entre 88 y 104 países y territorios presentaron cada año un total de entre 369 y 675 modificaciones de las previsiones establecidas. Durante ese período de diez años, 206 países y territorios en total presentaron al menos una previsión de una sustancia sicotrópica o modificaron una previsión establecida.

Cuadro 18. Previsiones de sustancias sicotrópicas y modificaciones recibidas de los países y territorios, 2014–2023

Año	*Previsiones*	*Países y territorios que presentaron previsiones*	*Modificaciones*	*Países y territorios que presentaron modificaciones*
2014	2 797	96	369	92
2015	2 690	92	513	98
2016	2 965	102	481	96
2017	3 192	104	398	88
2018	3 284	97	421	95
2019	3 700	97	500	90
2020	3 188	90	494	104
2021	2 983	94	607	90
2022	3 572	94	507	89
2023	3 680	94	675	94

140. Las sustancias respecto de las que los países y territorios presentaron el mayor número de previsiones actualizadas o de modificaciones de las previsiones establecidas figuraban también entre las sustancias objeto de fabricación y comercio más activos. Durante el período comprendido entre 2014 y 2023 se recibieron previsiones o modificaciones de las previsiones por parte de al menos un país o territorio respecto de un total de 146 sustancias, casi todas las incluidas en las Listas II, III y IV del Convenio de 1971. En el cuadro 19 figuran las sustancias que fueron objeto del mayor número de previsiones o modificaciones de las previsiones establecidas para 2023.

Cuadro 19. Sustancias sicotrópicas que fueron objeto del mayor número de previsiones o modificaciones de las previsiones por parte de los países y territorios para 2023

Sustancia	*Previsiones*	*Sustancia*	*Modificaciones*
Midazolam	100	Metilfenidato	42
Diazepam	100	Fenobarbital	23
Fenobarbital	99	Dexanfetamina	20
Clonazepam	95	Pentobarbital	18
Alprazolam	93	Buprenorfina	17

141. Para 2025, 70 países y territorios han presentado un total de 2.428 previsiones de sus necesidades de sustancias sicotrópicas. En el caso de los 144 países y territorios que no han facilitado previsiones actualizadas para 2025, se mantendrán las previsiones establecidas previamente para 2024. A diferencia del sistema de previsiones de estupefacientes, las existencias y el consumo de sustancias sicotrópicas comunicados con relación a un año no afectan las previsiones de esas sustancias para el año siguiente. En el cuadro 20 figuran las sustancias respecto de las que el mayor número de países y territorios actualizaron sus previsiones correspondientes a 2025.

Cuadro 20. Sustancias sicotrópicas que han sido objeto del mayor número de previsiones por los países y territorios para 2025

Sustancia	*Previsiones*
Diazepam	70
Midazolam	70
Clonazepam	68
Fenobarbital	67
Alprazolam	65

142. En los anexos publicados en línea figuran las previsiones para 2025 correspondientes a todos los países y territorios. Dado que los países y territorios pueden actualizar sus previsiones de sustancias sicotrópicas en cualquier momento, en el sitio web de la JIFE pueden consultarse las previsiones más actualizadas.

Tendencias de las cantidades de sustancias sicotrópicas previstas por los países y territorios

143. Dado que los países y territorios no están obligados a actualizar anualmente sus previsiones de sustancias sicotrópicas, estas no suelen cambiar significativamente de un año para otro. No obstante, como se indica en la sección anterior, muchos países modifican periódicamente sus evaluaciones globales a lo largo del año civil. El análisis que figura a continuación abarca las evaluaciones tal y como estaban a finales de 2023 y 2024 y para principios de 2025.

144. Para 2025, las sustancias sicotrópicas con las previsiones más altas, por peso bruto, son el fenobarbital (876,1 t), el GHB (238,0 t), el meprobamato (175,5 t), el metilfenidato (146,7 t), el diazepam (124,1 t), el pentobarbital (102,2 t), el zolpidem (92,8 t), la fentermina (62,2 t), el clordiazepóxido (57,8 t) y el barbital (50,9 t) (véase

Figura 15. Sustancias sicotrópicas que han sido objeto de las mayores previsiones, por peso bruto, 2023–2025

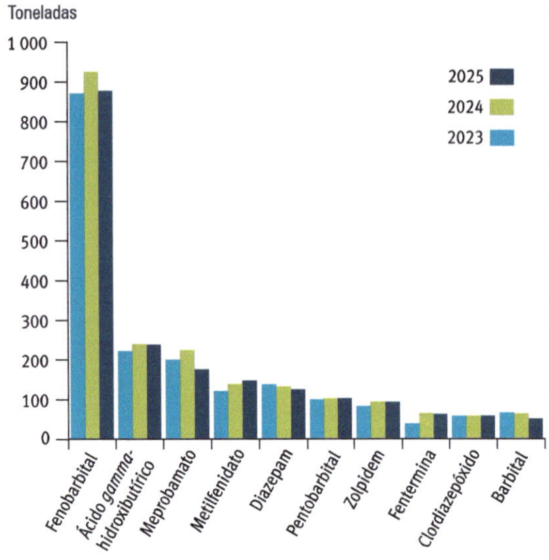

Figura 16. Sustancias sicotrópicas que han sido objeto de las mayores previsiones, por S-DDD, 2023–2025

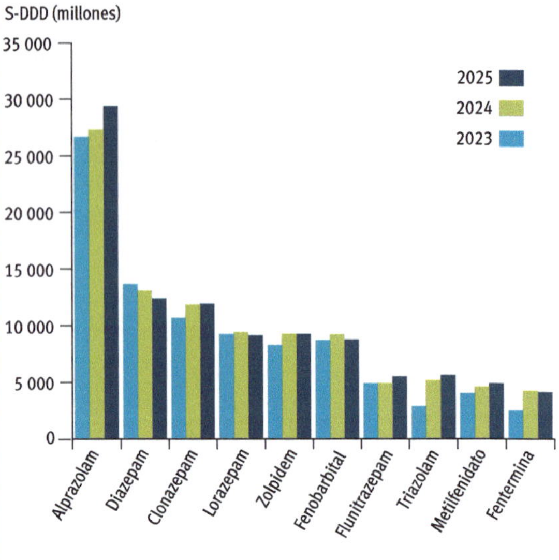

la figura 15). Las previsiones de fenobarbital para 2025 han disminuido con respecto a las 923,8 t de 2024. Del mismo modo, las previsiones de meprobamato, diazepam y barbital han disminuido en comparación con años anteriores. Las previsiones de metilfenidato han aumentado en aproximadamente 10 t. Además, las previsiones de fentermina para 2025 casi se han duplicado en comparación con las de 2023, impulsadas en gran medida por el aumento de las cantidades previstas por México y los Estados Unidos.

145. Las sustancias sicotrópicas para las que se han presentado mayores previsiones en términos de dosis (S-DDD) son muy distintas de aquellas para las que se han presentado mayores previsiones expresadas en términos de peso bruto. Para 2025, las sustancias para las que se han presentado mayores previsiones en términos de S-DDD son el alprazolam (29.400 millones de S-DDD), el diazepam (12.400 millones de S-DDD), el clonazepam (11.900 millones de S-DDD), el zolpidem (9.300 millones de S-DDD), el lorazepam (9.200 millones de S-DDD), el fenobarbital (8.800 millones de S-DDD), el triazolam (5.600 millones de S-DDD), el flunitrazepam (5.500 millones de S-DDD), el metilfenidato (4.900 millones de S-DDD) y la fentermina (4.100 millones de S-DDD).

146. Como puede verse en la figura 16, las previsiones de alprazolam a nivel mundial son más del doble que las del diazepam, la segunda sustancia con mayores previsiones. En particular, las previsiones de alprazolam para 2025 han aumentado en 2.700 millones de S-DDD en comparación con las de 2023. Asimismo, las previsiones de triazolam para 2025 se han duplicado en comparación con las de 2023. Tanto en términos de peso bruto como de S-DDD, las previsiones de diazepam han disminuido. Las demás sustancias con mayores previsiones en términos de S-DDD solo mostraron ligeros cambios y fluctuaciones entre 2023 y 2025.

About the International Narcotics Control Board

The International Narcotics Control Board (INCB) is an independent and quasi-judicial control organ, established by treaty, that monitors the implementation of the international drug control treaties. It had predecessors under the former drug control treaties as far back as the time of the League of Nations.

Composition

INCB consists of 13 members who are elected by the Economic and Social Council and who serve in their personal capacity, not as government representatives. Three members with medical, pharmacological or pharmaceutical experience are elected from a list of persons nominated by the World Health Organization (WHO) and 10 members are elected from a list of persons nominated by Governments. Members of the Board are persons who, by their competence, impartiality and disinterestedness, command general confidence. The Council, in consultation with INCB, makes all arrangements necessary to ensure the full technical independence of the Board in carrying out its functions. INCB has a secretariat that assists it in the exercise of its treaty-related functions. The INCB secretariat is an administrative entity of the United Nations Office on Drugs and Crime, but it reports solely to the Board on matters of substance. INCB closely collaborates with the Office in the framework of arrangements approved by the Council in its resolution 1991/48. INCB also cooperates with other international bodies concerned with drug control, including not only the Council and its Commission on Narcotic Drugs, but also the relevant specialized agencies of the United Nations, particularly WHO. It also cooperates with bodies outside the United Nations system, especially the International Criminal Police Organization (INTERPOL) and the World Customs Organization (WCO).

Functions

The functions of INCB are laid down in the following treaties: the Single Convention on Narcotic Drugs of 1961 as amended by the 1972 Protocol; the Convention on Psychotropic Substances of 1971; and the United Nations Convention against Illicit Traffic in Narcotic Drugs and Psychotropic Substances of 1988. Broadly speaking, INCB deals with the following:

(a) As regards the licit manufacture of, trade in and use of drugs, INCB endeavours, in cooperation with Governments, to ensure that adequate supplies of drugs are available for medical and scientific uses and that the diversion of drugs from licit sources to illicit channels does not occur. INCB also monitors Governments' control over chemicals used in the illicit manufacture of drugs and assists them in preventing the diversion of those chemicals into illicit traffic;

(b) As regards the illicit manufacture of, trafficking in and use of drugs, INCB identifies weaknesses in national and international control systems and contributes to correcting such situations. INCB is also responsible for assessing chemicals used in the illicit manufacture of drugs in order to determine whether they should be placed under international control.

In the discharge of its responsibilities, INCB:

(a) Administers a system of estimates for narcotic drugs and a voluntary assessment system for psychotropic substances and monitors licit activities involving drugs through a statistical returns system, with a view to assisting Governments in achieving, inter alia, a balance between supply and demand;

(b) Monitors and promotes measures taken by Governments to prevent the diversion of substances frequently used in the illicit manufacture of narcotic drugs and psychotropic substances and assesses such substances to determine whether there is a need for changes in the scope of control of Tables I and II of the 1988 Convention;

(c) Analyses information provided by Governments, United Nations bodies, specialized agencies and other competent international organizations, with a view to ensuring that the provisions of the international drug control treaties are adequately carried out by Governments, and recommends remedial measures;

(d) Maintains a permanent dialogue with Governments to assist them in complying with their obligations under the international drug control treaties and, to that end, recommends, where appropriate, technical or financial assistance of the provision.

INCB is called upon to ask for explanations in the event of apparent violations of the treaties, to propose appropriate remedial measures to Governments that are not fully applying the provisions of the treaties or are encountering difficulties in applying them and, where necessary, to assist Governments in overcoming such difficulties. If, however, INCB notes that the measures necessary to remedy a serious situation have not been taken, it may bring the matter to the attention of the parties concerned, the Commission on Narcotic Drugs and the Economic and Social Council. As a last resort, the treaties empower INCB to recommend to parties that they stop importing drugs from a defaulting country, exporting drugs to it or both. In all cases, INCB acts in close cooperation with Governments.

INCB assists national administrations in meeting their obligations under the conventions. To that end, it proposes and participates in regional training seminars and programmes for drug control administrators.

Reports

The international drug control treaties require INCB to prepare an annual report on its work. The annual report contains an analysis of the drug control situation worldwide so that Governments are kept aware of existing and potential situations that may endanger the objectives of the international drug control treaties. INCB draws the attention of Governments to gaps and weaknesses in national control and in treaty compliance; it also makes suggestions and recommendations for improvements at both the national and international levels. The annual report is based on information provided by Governments to INCB, United Nations entities and other organizations. It also uses information provided through other international organizations, such as INTERPOL and WCO, as well as regional organizations.

The annual report of INCB is supplemented by detailed technical reports. They contain data on the licit movement of narcotic drugs and psychotropic substances required for medical and scientific purposes, together with an analysis of those data by INCB. Those data are required for the proper functioning of the system of control over the licit movement of narcotic drugs and psychotropic substances, including preventing their diversion to illicit channels. Moreover, under the provisions of article 12 of the 1988 Convention, INCB reports annually to the Commission on Narcotic Drugs on the implementation of that article. That report, which gives an account of the results of the monitoring of precursors and of the chemicals frequently used in the illicit manufacture of narcotic drugs and psychotropic substances, is also published as a supplement to the annual report.

Le rôle de l'Organe international de contrôle des stupéfiants

L'Organe international de contrôle des stupéfiants (OICS) est un organe de contrôle indépendant et quasi-judiciaire, créé par traité, qui surveille l'application des traités internationaux relatifs au contrôle des drogues. Il a été précédé par d'autres organes qui, du temps de la Société des Nations, déjà œuvraient dans ce domaine en vertu des précédents traités relatifs au contrôle des drogues.

Composition de l'OICS

L'OICS se compose de 13 membres élus par le Conseil économique et social, qui siègent à titre personnel et non en qualité de représentants de leur pays. Trois membres ayant l'expérience de la médecine, de la pharmacologie ou de la pharmacie sont choisis sur une liste de personnes désignées par l'Organisation mondiale de la santé (OMS) et 10 membres sur une liste de personnes désignées par les gouvernements. Les membres de l'OICS doivent être des personnes qui, par leur compétence, leur impartialité et leur désintéressement, inspirent la confiance générale. Le Conseil prend, en consultation avec l'OICS, toutes les dispositions nécessaires pour assurer la pleine indépendance technique de ce dernier dans l'exercice de ses fonctions. L'OICS a un secrétariat chargé de l'aider dans l'exercice des fonctions qui lui incombent au titre des traités. Ce secrétariat est une unité administrative de l'Office des Nations Unies contre la drogue et le crime, mais, pour les questions de fond, il en réfère exclusivement à l'OICS. Ce dernier collabore étroitement avec l'Office dans le cadre des dispositions approuvées par le Conseil économique et social dans sa résolution 1991/48. L'OICS collabore également avec d'autres organismes internationaux qui s'occupent aussi du contrôle des drogues. Au nombre de ces organismes figurent non seulement le Conseil et sa Commission des stupéfiants, mais aussi les institutions spécialisées des Nations Unies compétentes en la matière, en particulier l'OMS. L'OICS coopère également avec des organismes qui n'appartiennent pas au système des Nations Unies, en particulier l'Organisation internationale de police criminelle (OIPC/Interpol) et l'Organisation mondiale des douanes (OMD).

Fonctions de l'OICS

Les fonctions de l'OICS sont énoncées dans les traités suivants: la Convention unique sur les stupéfiants de 1961, telle que modifiée par le Protocole de 1972; la Convention sur les substances psychotropes de 1971; et la Convention des Nations Unies contre le trafic illicite de stupéfiants et de substances psychotropes de 1988. En gros, les fonctions de l'OICS sont les suivantes:

a) En ce qui concerne la fabrication, le commerce et l'usage licites des drogues, l'OICS, agissant en coopération avec les gouvernements, s'efforce de faire en sorte que soient disponibles en quantité suffisante les drogues requises à des fins médicales et scientifiques et que les drogues ne soient pas détournées des sources licites vers les circuits illicites. L'OICS surveille également comment les gouvernements contrôlent les produits chimiques utilisés dans la fabrication illicite des drogues et les aide à prévenir le détournement de ces produits vers le trafic illicite;

b) En ce qui concerne la fabrication, le trafic et l'usage illicites des drogues, l'OICS identifie les lacunes qui existent dans les systèmes de contrôle national et international et contribue à y remédier. Il est également chargé d'évaluer les produits chimiques utilisés dans la fabrication illicite des drogues afin de déterminer s'il y a lieu de les placer sous contrôle international;

Pour s'acquitter des tâches qui lui sont imparties, l'OICS:

a) Administre un régime d'évaluations pour les stupéfiants et un système volontaire de prévisions pour les substances psychotropes et surveille les activités licites relatives aux drogues à l'aide d'un système de rapports statistiques, pour aider les gouvernements à réaliser, notamment, un équilibre entre l'offre et la demande;

b) Suit et encourage les mesures prises par les gouvernements pour prévenir le détournement de substances fréquemment utilisées dans la fabrication illicite de stupéfiants et de substances psychotropes, et évalue les substances de ce type afin de déterminer s'il y a lieu de modifier le champ d'application des Tableaux I et II de la Convention de 1988;

c) Analyse les renseignements fournis par les gouvernements, les organes de l'Organisation des Nations Unies, les institutions spécialisées et d'autres organisations internationales compétentes, afin de veiller à ce que les dispositions des traités internationaux relatifs au contrôle des drogues soient appliquées de façon appropriée par les gouvernements, et recommande, le cas échéant, des mesures correctives;

d) Entretient un dialogue permanent avec les gouvernements pour les aider à s'acquitter de leurs obligations en vertu des traités internationaux relatifs au contrôle des drogues et, à cette fin, recommande, le cas échéant, la prestation d'une assistance technique ou financière.

L'OICS est appelé à demander des explications en cas de violation apparente des traités, à proposer aux gouvernements qui n'en appliquent pas entièrement les dispositions, ou rencontrent des difficultés à les appliquer, les mesures correctives appropriées et à les aider, le cas échéant, à surmonter ces difficultés. Si, toutefois, l'OICS constate que les mesures propres à remédier à une situation grave n'ont pas été prises, il peut porter le problème à l'attention des parties intéressées, de la Commission des stupéfiants et du Conseil économique et social. En dernier recours, les traités autorisent l'OICS à recommander aux parties d'arrêter l'importation ou l'exportation de drogues, ou les deux, en provenance ou à destination du pays défaillant. Dans toutes circonstances, l'OICS agit en étroite collaboration avec les gouvernements.

L'OICS aide les administrations nationales à s'acquitter de leurs obligations en vertu des conventions. Pour ce faire, il propose des séminaires et stages de formation régionaux à l'intention des administrateurs chargés du contrôle des drogues et y participe.

Rapports de l'OICS

En vertu des traités internationaux relatifs au contrôle des drogues, l'OICS doit établir un rapport annuel sur ses activités. Ce rapport analyse la situation mondiale en matière de contrôle des drogues et permet ainsi de tenir les autorités nationales informées des problèmes qui se posent aujourd'hui ou risquent de se poser demain et qui sont de nature à compromettre la réalisation des objectifs des traités internationaux relatifs au contrôle des drogues. L'OICS appelle l'attention des États sur les lacunes et les insuffisances constatées dans le domaine du contrôle national et de l'application des traités. En outre, il suggère et recommande des améliorations aux niveaux international et national. Le rapport est fondé sur les renseignements communiqués par les gouvernements à l'OICS, ainsi qu'aux autres organes et organismes des Nations Unies. Il s'appuie également sur des informations fournies par l'intermédiaire d'autres organisations internationales, telles que l'OIPC/Interpol et l'OMD, ainsi que des organisations régionales.

Le rapport annuel de l'OICS est complété par des rapports techniques détaillés qui présentent des données concernant le mouvement licite des stupéfiants et des substances psychotropes requis à des fins médicales et scientifiques ainsi que l'analyse par l'OICS de ces données. Ces dernières sont nécessaires au bon fonctionnement des mécanismes de contrôle du mouvement licite des stupéfiants et des substances psychotropes, ainsi qu'à la prévention de leur détournement vers les circuits illicites. De plus, en vertu des dispositions de l'article 12 de la Convention de 1988, l'OICS fait rapport chaque année à la Commission des stupéfiants sur l'application dudit article. Ce rapport, qui fait état des résultats du contrôle des précurseurs et des produits chimiques fréquemment utilisés dans la fabrication illicite de stupéfiants et de substances psychotropes, est également publié comme supplément au rapport annuel.

Información sobre la Junta Internacional de Fiscalización de Estupefacientes

La Junta Internacional de Fiscalización de Estupefacientes (JIFE) es un órgano de fiscalización independiente y cuasi judicial, establecido por un tratado, que visila la aplicación de los tratados de fiscalización internacional de drogas. Sus predecesores en virtud de los anteriores tratados de fiscalización de drogas datan de la época de la Sociedad de Naciones.

Composición

La JIFE está constituida por 13 miembros elegidos por el Consejo Económico y Social que desempeñan sus funciones a título personal y no como representantes de los gobiernos. Tres de sus miembros, con experiencia en el campo de la medicina, la farmacología o la farmacia se seleccionan de una lista de candidatos presentada por la Organización Mundial de la Salud (OMS) y los otros diez de una lista de candidatos propuesta por los gobiernos. Los miembros de la JIFE son personas que gozan de la confianza general por su competencia, imparcialidad e independencia. El Consejo, en consulta con la JIFE, lleva a cabo todos los arreglos necesarios para asegurar la plena independencia técnica de la Junta en el desempeño de sus funciones. La JIFE cuenta con una secretaría que la asiste en el ejercicio de las funciones que le corresponden en virtud de los tratados. La secretaría de la JIFE es una entidad administrativa de la Oficina de las Naciones Unidas contra la Droga y el Delito, pero presenta sus informes sobre cuestiones de fondo únicamente a la Junta. La JIFE colabora estrechamente con la Oficina en el marco de los acuerdos aprobados por el Consejo en su resolución 1991/48. La JIFE colabora también con otros órganos internacionales relacionados con la fiscalización de drogas, entre los que se incluyen no sólo el Consejo y la Comisión de Estupefacientes, sino también los organismos especializados pertinentes de las Naciones Unidas, en particular la OMS. También colabora con órganos que no forman parte del sistema de las Naciones Unidas, en especial con la Organización Internacional de Policía Criminal (Interpol) y con la Organización Mundial de Aduanas (OMA).

Funciones

Las funciones de la JIFE están consagradas en los siguientes tratados: la Convención Única sobre Estupefacientes de 1961, enmendada por el Protocolo de 1972; el Convenio sobre Sustancias Sicotrópicas de 1971; y la Convención de las Naciones Unidas contra el Tráfico Ilícito de Estupefacientes y Sustancias Sicotrópicas de 1988. En términos generales, la JIFE se ocupa de lo siguiente:

a) En relación con la fabricación, el comercio y el uso lícitos de drogas, la JIFE, en cooperación con los gobiernos, procura asegurar que haya suministros de drogas adecuados para fines médicos y científicos y que no se produzcan desviaciones de drogas de fuentes lícitas a canales ilícitos. La JIFE también vigila la fiscalización que aplican los gobiernos a los productos químicos utilizados en la fabricación ilícita de drogas y les presta asistencia para prevenir la desviación de esos productos químicos hacia el tráfico ilícito;

b) En relación con la fabricación, el tráfico y el uso ilícitos de drogas, la JIFE determina las deficiencias de los sistemas de fiscalización nacionales e internacionales y contribuye a corregir esas situaciones. La JIFE también tiene a su cargo la evaluación de los productos químicos utilizados en la fabricación ilícita de drogas, a fin de determinar si deben ser sometidos a fiscalización internacional.

En cumplimiento de esas obligaciones, la JIFE:

a) Administra un sistema de previsiones de las necesidades de estupefacientes y un sistema de presentación voluntaria de previsiones de las necesidades de sustancias sicotrópicas, y supervisa las actividades lícitas con drogas mediante un sistema de información estadística, con miras a ayudar a los gobiernos a lograr, entre otras cosas, un equilibrio entre la oferta y la demanda;

b) Vigila y promueve las medidas tomadas por los gobiernos para impedir la desviación de sustancias utilizadas frecuentemente en la fabricación ilícita de estupefacientes y sustancias sicotrópicas, y evalúa tales sustancias para determinar si es necesario modificar el ámbito de la fiscalización aplicada en virtud de los Cuadros I y II de la Convención de 1988;

c) Analiza la información proporcionada por los gobiernos, los órganos de las Naciones Unidas, los organismos especializados y otras organizaciones internacionales competentes, con miras a velar por que los gobiernos cumplan adecuadamente las disposiciones de los tratados internacionales sobre fiscalización de drogas, y recomienda las medidas correctivas necesarias;

d) Mantiene un diálogo permanente con los gobiernos para ayudarlos a cumplir las obligaciones que les imponen los tratados de fiscalización internacional de drogas y recomienda, cuando procede, que se proporcione asistencia técnica o financiera con esa finalidad.

La JIFE debe pedir explicaciones en casos de violaciones aparentes de los tratados, a fin de proponer las medidas correctivas apropiadas a los gobiernos que no estén aplicando plenamente las disposiciones de los tratados, o que tropiecen con dificultades para aplicarlas y, cuando sea necesario, prestar asistencia a los gobiernos para superar esas dificultades. Ahora bien, si la JIFE observa que no se han tomado las medidas necesarias para remediar una situación grave, puede señalar la cuestión a la atención de las partes interesadas, la Comisión de Estupefacientes y el Consejo Económico y Social. Los tratados facultan a la JIFE, como último recurso, para recomendar a las partes que dejen de importar drogas del país que haya incurrido en falta, o que no exporten drogas a ese país, o ambas cosas. En todos los casos, la JIFE actúa en estrecha cooperación con los gobiernos.

La JIFE presta asistencia a las administraciones públicas de los países para que cumplan las obligaciones que les corresponden de conformidad con los convenios y convenciones. A ese fin, la JIFE propone programas y seminarios de capacitación regional dirigidos a funcionarios de las administraciones que trabajan en la fiscalización de drogas y participa en dichos programas y seminarios.

Informes

Los tratados internacionales de fiscalización de drogas exigen que la JIFE prepare un informe anual sobre la labor que realiza. En el informe anual figura un análisis de la situación mundial de la fiscalización de drogas a fin de que los gobiernos tengan conocimiento de la existencia y las posibles situaciones que pueden poner en peligro los objetivos de los tratados internacionales de fiscalización de drogas. La JIFE señala a la atención de los gobiernos las lagunas y deficiencias que existen en la fiscalización nacional de drogas y en el cumplimiento de los tratados; asimismo hace sugerencias y recomendaciones con el fin de lograr mejoras tanto en el plano nacional como internacional. El informe anual se basa en la información que proporcionan los gobiernos a la JIFE, entidades de las Naciones Unidas y otras organizaciones. También se utiliza información que se obtiene por mediación de otras organizaciones internacionales, como la Interpol y la OMA, así como de organizaciones regionales.

El informe anual de la JIFE se complementa con informes técnicos detallados en los que figuran datos sobre el movimiento lícito de estupefacientes y sustancias sicotrópicas utilizados para fines médicos y científicos, junto con un análisis que realiza la JIFE de esos datos. Los datos son necesarios para el funcionamiento adecuado del sistema de fiscalización del movimiento lícito de estupefacientes y sustancias sicotrópicas, incluida su desviación a canales ilícitos. Además, de conformidad con lo dispuesto en el artículo 12 de la Convención de 1988, la JIFE informa anualmente a la Comisión de Estupefacientes sobre la aplicación de este artículo. Dicho informe, en el que se recogen los resultados de la vigilancia de los precursores y los productos químicos que se utilizan con frecuencia en la fabricación ilícita de estupefacientes y sustancias sicotrópicas, se publica también como complemento del informe anual.